Aids to Postgraduate Surgery

Aids to Postgraduate Surgery

Meirion Thomas

M.B., B.S., M.R.C.P., F.R.C.S.,
Lecturer in Surgery, Institute of Cancer Research,
Royal Marsden Hospital, Sutton, Surrey.

John S. Belstead

M.B., Ch.B., F.R.C.S. (Edin)
Senior Registrar in Orthopaedic Surgery,
Westminster Hospital, London

CHURCHILL LIVINGSTONE
EDINBURGH LONDON AND NEW YORK 1976

CHURCHILL LIVINGSTONE

Medical Division of Longman Group Limited

Distributed in the United States of America by Longman Inc., 19 West 44th Street, New York, N.Y. 10036 and by associated companies, branches and representatives throughout the world.

© Longman Group Limited 1976

First Edition 1976
Reprinted 1978

ISBN 0 443 01511 2

Library of Congress Cataloging in Publication Data

Thomas, Meirion.
    Aids to postgraduate surgery.

    Bibliography: p
    1. Surgery. I. Belstead, John S., joint author.
II. Title. DNLM: 1. Surgery. WO100 T459a
RD31.T53   617   76-16565

Printed in Hong Kong
by Hong Kong Printing Press (1977) Ltd

Preface

It is the prerequisite of the surgeon that, apart from basic surgical ability, he must be able to appraise the relative merits of different patterns of management. The surgical examinations are particularly biased in this direction.

The student will gain most of his knowledge from textbooks. He will then complement this knowledge with experience, discussion, the attendance of postgraduate lectures and an extensive perusal of many journals.

Having recently experienced the practical problems of studying for the F.R.C.S. examination we felt there was a need for a text that would at least attempt to review the most recent opinions and developments in surgery and guide the student to some key references where more detailed considerations may be sought. The search for references can be time-consuming and tedious. The references selected have been drawn wherever possible from the more commonly available journals and we hope that they will be of benefit. References listed under further reading are not tabulated in any order of merit but in alphabetical order of authors' surnames.

The selection of topics is based mainly upon areas of current controversy in surgery and areas of knowledge largely contained only in journals.

Although this text is intended mainly for the postgraduate student, we hope that senior medical students will find it of benefit.

Acknowledgements

We wish to thank the many colleagues who have helped in the preparation of this book by their advice and criticism.

Our thanks are also due to Miss Caroline Edwards and Miss Elaine Etgert for their patience and hard work in typing and retyping the drafts.

Gratitude must also be expressed to our wives and families for their tolerance in the months of writing.

Contents

Oesophago-gastro-duodenoscopy

INDICATIONS

1. Ideally, as a preliminary to surgery to the oesophagus, stomach or duodenum
2. In barium negative dyspepsia
3. In acute gastro-intestinal haemorrhage.
    The most accurate method of diagnosis
    Bleeding point visualised in 90% patients
    Patients with known ulcers may bleed from other sites, e.g. acute erosions, oesophagitis
    Radiology limited in the diagnosis of superficial lesions or stomal ulcers
    No evidence that endoscopy precipitates further haemorrhage
4. In the investigation of suspected stomal ulceration
    Surgical distortion produces confusing radiological appearance
    Radiology detects only 50% of stomal ulcers and makes false positive diagnoses
    Endoscopy detects 90% of stomal ulcers
    (Non-absorbable suture causing stomal ulceration can be removed by biopsy forceps)
5. For assessment (including biopsy) of radiologically diagnosed gastric ulcers especially those in the antral region
6. To detect gastric carcinoma developing after surgery for benign conditions
    Carcinoma in the gastric stump is significantly more common than carcinoma in the non-operated stomach
    Average time between surgery and development of carcinoma is 23 years
    Carcinoma develops usually at the site of anastomosis and is thought to be related to bile-induced atrophic gastritis
    Supporting evidence is that carcinoma develops more commonly after Polya gastrectomy and gastrojejunostomy than Bilroth I gastrectomy.
    (Experimentally, atrophic gastritis after Polya gastrectomy is reversed when the anastomosis is converted to Roux-Y, so preventing bile reflux)

FURTHER READING

Cotton, P.B., Rosenberg, M.T., Axon, A.R.T., Davis, M., Pierce, J.W., Price, A.B., Stevenson, G.W. & Waldran, R. (1973) Diagnostic yield of fibre-optic endoscopy in the operated stomach. *British Journal of Surgery*, **60**, 629-632.
Cotton, P. B., Rosenberg, M.T., Waldran, R.P.L. & Axon, A.R.T. (1973) Early endoscopy of oesophagus, stomach and duodenal bulb in patients with haematemesis and melaena. *British Medical Journal*, **2**, 505-509.

Endoscopic retrograde cholangiopancreatography (ERCP)

1. Performed via side-viewing duodenoscope
2. Contra-indicated in recent acute pancreatitis and Australian Antigenaemia (possible method of transmission of AA)
3. Has been performed via afferent loop of Polya gastrectomy. Previous sphincterotomy or sphincteroplasty facilitate cannulation of papilla
4. Oesophagus, stomach and duodenum should be carefully scrutinised for associated abnormalities, e.g. jaundice caused by secondary deposits at porta hepatis from gastric primary. Duodenal loop should be fully examined for distortion, mucosal ulceration, infiltration or diverticulae

INDICATIONS

1. Retrograde cholangiography in the investigation of jaundice or recurrent jaundice
   i. In this situation oral or i.v. cholangiography may be of little value
   ii. Has the advantage over percutaneous transhepatic cholangiography which should only be performed pre-operatively
   iii. May show the following abnormalities:
      a. A filling defect in the biliary tree
      b. A dilated CBD
      c. A failure of contrast to reach the gall bladder
      d. The site and extent of stricture of CBD
      e. Stenosis of biliary tree (by factors in the lumen, in the wall and outside the wall)
2. Retrograde pancreatography in the investigation of pancreatic disease
   i. Pancreatic carcinoma may completely obstruct main pancreatic duct
   ii. In chronic or relapsing pancreatitis surgical intervention may depend on assessment of the following abnormalities of the main pancreatic duct:
      a. Minor calibre variations
      b. Major calibre variations (beading)
      c. Stricture with proximal dilation
      d. Complete obstruction

COMPLICATIONS

1. Febrile reactions, acute cholangitis, and septicaemia associated with an obstructed, infected biliary tree
2. Transmission of serum hepatitis
3. Acute pancreatitis. Elevation of serum and urinary amylase occurs frequently but clinical pancreatitis is rare. Associated especially with contrast material filling the acini (parenchymography) as well as the pancreatic ductal system

Colonoscopy

1. Can be used per anum in the intact or resected colon; via a terminal colostomy, a loop colostomy, or an ileostomy
2. In the intact colon particular difficulty may be experienced negotiating the apex of the sigmoid loop or splenic flexure. A greater length of bowel can be more easily visualised in the resected colon or via a colostomy
3. The sigmoid colon is difficult to assess radiologically due to segments of colon overlying each other. Colonoscopy is especially useful in this region

INDICATIONS

1. In the search for adenomas or early malignant lesions in symptomatic patients with negative or equivocal radiology
2. In the search for adenomas, metachronous carcinoma or suture line recurrence in patients who have previously undergone resection for carcinoma
3. For assessment and biopsy of radiologically-suggestive inflammatory disease of colon, e.g. a localised colonic segment of Crohn's disease
4. To estimate the extent of colonic involvement in ulcerative colitis. Patients with radiologically defined distal colitis may have much more extensive involvement confirmed on colonoscopy
5. To confirm or exclude possible carcinoma suggested radiologically in a segment of diverticular disease
6. To perform polypectomy using colonoscopic diathermy snare
Preferable to laparotomy, colotomy and surgical polypectomy in the management of polyps inaccessible to the rigid sigmoidoscope

FURTHER READING

Williams, C. & Teague, R. (1973) Progress report. Colonoscopy. *Gut,* **14**, 990-1003.

Carcinoma of oesophagus

OESOPHAGEAL SUBDIVISIONS
1. Upper third: From crico-pharyngeus to aortic arch
   - i. True cervical oesophagus
   - ii. Supra-aortic oesophagus
2. Middle third: From aortic arch to inferior pulmonary vein
3. Lower third: From inferior pulmonary vein to gastro-oesophageal junction
   - i. Supra-diaphragmatic oesophagus
   - ii. Abdominal oesophagus

SPREAD OF OESOPHAGEAL CARCINOMA
1. Direct spread
   - i. Submucosal spread
       - Longitudinal or circumferential
   - ii. Transmural
       - Recurrent laryngeal nerve (usually the left)
       - Trachea
       - Bronchus (oesophagobronchial fistula)
       - Aorta.
       - Crura of diaphragm
2. Lymphatic spread
   - i. Intramural lymphatic permeation and embolisation. Satellite growths found microscopically well beyond macroscopic limit of growth, so that a clearance of 6 cm of 'normal' oesophagus is required. Access to a sufficient length of 'normal' oesophagus dictates the surgical approach and forms the rational basis for total oesophagectomy
   - ii. Upper third: Cervical lymph nodes
     Middle third: Hilar and subcarinal nodes
     Then to paratracheal and cervical nodes, or to coeliac nodes
     Lower third: Coeliac nodes

(This pattern of lymphatic spread and the proximity of vital structures dictates that radical surgery is possible only for growths in the lower third of oesophagus).

3. Blood borne spread
   - Liver
   - Bone
   - Skin

SURGERY TO CARCINOMA LOWER THIRD OESOPHAGUS

1. Tumours below the diaphragm (unless there is peritoneal or abdominal visceral spread) can be excised radically through a left thoracoabdominal approach together with stomach, spleen, tail of pancreas, omenta, the regional lymphatic field and restoring continuity by oesophago-jejunal anastomosis en-Roux, or oesophagogastrostomy.
2. Carcinoma above the diaphragm should be excised by the Lewis-Tanner Operation (the two-stage procedure). Access to sufficient length of 'normal' oesophagus is not possible through a left thoracoabdominal approach. The stomach is mobilised on the right gastric and gastroepiploic arteries at laparotomy, and Kocher procedure and pyloromyotomy are performed. Through a right thoracotomy, the tumour and lower oesophagus are mobilised and the stomach is drawn into the chest. The tumour with adequate clearance of 'normal' oesophagus and the proximal stomach are resected and continuity is restored by oesophagogastric anastomosis.

SURGERY TO CARCINOMA MIDDLE THIRD OESOPHAGUS

1. For carcinoma in the lower half of the middle third of oesophagus, the Lewis-Tanner Operation can be performed.
2. When a carcinoma of the upper half of the middle third is removed by the two-stage procedure, then to allow adequate clearance above the tumour, the oesophagogastric anastomosis will have to be performed high in the superior mediastinum. The dangers of such a difficult anastomosis can be reduced by a three stage total oesophagectomy. The third stage involves the mobilisation of the cervical oesophagus through a right supraclavicular incision; the delivery of the oesophagus into the neck wound; oesophagectomy with closure of the oesophagogastric junction; and restoration of continuity by anastomosing the cervical oesophagus to gastric fundus.

TREATMENT OF CARCINOMA OF UPPER THIRD OESOPHAGUS

1. The three stage total oesophagectomy
2. Radiotherapy

THE PLACE OF RADIOTHERAPY IN CARCINOMA OF OESOPHAGUS

1. It has been claimed that megavoltage irradiation to squamous carcinoma of oesophagus offers a better 5-year survival than surgery. One of the reasons for this was the absence of treatment mortality following irradiation. However the surgical series used for comparison with radiotherapy was collected between 1948 and 1963, since when improvement in techniques will have improved operative mortality. Adenocarcinoma of oesophagus (10% of total) arising from oesophageal mucous glands is radioresistant.

    Pearson, J.G. (1971) The value of radiotherapy in the management of squamous oesophageal cancer. *British Journal of Surgery,* **58,** 794-798.

2. Postoperative radiotherapy to known residual tumour may improve the survival rate. However, if the stoma lies within the field of irradiation, stomal necrosis may occur. In the three stage total oesophagectomy, the stoma is outside the field of irradiation, allowing safe irradiation of hilar and carinal nodes.

TREATMENT OF UNRESECTABLE CARCINOMA OF OESOPHAGUS

About 50% of carcinomata of middle third of oesophagus are unresectable. Intubation of oesophageal carcinoma has given discouraging results:
1. Retrosternal pain and discomfort
2. Only partial relief of dysphagia. In one series 50% of patients could swallow liquids only and did not leave hospital
3. Repeated obstruction of endo-oesophageal tube requiring clearance through an oesophagoscope
4. Oesophageal perforation during dilation and intubation of carcinoma
5. Erosion of the oesophageal wall by the tube resulting in perforation or fistula formation

Subcutaneous or retrosternal bypass of unresectable carcinoma by colon, jejunum or stomach has been reported.
1. Operative mortality of 28.3% in an unselected series
2. 71.7% of patients discharged from hospital
3. Of these, 66% could eat a normal diet and 34% could eat soft foods only
4. Average survival was four months after operation

Celestin, L.R. (1959) Permanent intubation of inoperable cancer of the oesophagus and cardia. *Annals of the Royal College of Surgeons of England,* **25,** 165-170.

Ong, G.B. (1975) Unresectable carcinoma of the oesophagus. *Annals of the Royal College of Surgeons of England,* **56,** 3-14.

FURTHER READING

Leigh Collis, J. (1971) Surgical treatment of carcinoma of the oesophagus and cardia. *British Journal of Surgery,* **58,** 801-804.

McKeown, K.C. (1972) Trends in oesophageal resection for carcinoma with special reference to total oesophagectomy. *Annals of the Royal College of Surgeons of England,* **51,** 213-239.

McKeown, K.C. (1973) Carcinoma of the oesophagus. In *Recent Advances in Surgery,* ed. Selwyn Taylor. Ch.6, pp. 133-165. Edinburgh and London: Churchill Livingstone.

Hiatus hernia

CLASSIFICATION

1. Paraoesophageal hernia

The competent oesophago-gastric junction (OGJ) may lie above or below the diaphragm, but the apex of the hernia is formed by a pouch of stomach which herniates alongside the lower oesophagus.

2. Sliding hernia

Where an incompetent OGJ forms the apex of the hernia and where the complications of reflux oesophagitis, stricture and oesophageal shortening are seen.

THEORIES OF AETIOLOGY

1. Primarily an anatomical abnormality in the obese middle aged where weak ligaments and muscles fail to anchor the OGJ in its infra diaphragmatic position. The stomach is then displaced into the posterior mediastinum by raised intra-abdominal pressure.
2. The result of excessive traction by oesophageal longitudinal muscle hauling the OGJ into the posterior mediastinum. This functional abnormality may be caused by abnormal neuromuscular co-ordination or by gastro-intestinal hormonal imbalance, factors which may eventually correlate with the high incidence of obesity, cholelithiasis, gastric hypermobility and hypersection in these patients.

FACTORS CONTRIBUTING TO OGJ COMPETENCE

1. A length of intra-abdominal oesophagus which implants obliquely into the stomach forming an acute angle with the fundus
2. The presence of an intrinsic lower oesophageal sphincter
3. A compressed abdominal oesophagus, the result of its lumen being at intrathoracic (negative) pressure lying in the positive pressure of the abdomen
4. The support given to the abdominal oesophagus by the right crus of diaphragm

CONSERVATIVE TREATMENT

85% of symptomatic patients can be treated successfully:
1. Weight loss. Sleep propped upright
2. No food or drink after early evening
3. Preparations to protect oesophageal mucosa, e.g. antacids, silicones and alginates

INDICATIONS FOR SURGERY

1. Failure to respond to conservative management
2. Peptic stricture
3. Oesophageal ulceration discreet enough to see on barium swallow
4. Respiratory complications from the reflux of oesophageal contents into the trachea. Productive cough, lung abscess, or even empyema can occur
5. Significant anaemia and haemorrhage
6. A huge hiatus hernia causing post-prandial cardio-respiratory distress
7. During laparotomy for concomitant conditions (e.g. duodenal ulceration, cholelithiasis)

SURGICAL RELIEF OF SYMPTOMS

All the surgical procedures described are designed to achieve one or more of the following objectives:
1. Closure of hiatus by apposition of the two limbs of right crus
2. Anchoring of the OGJ in its sub-diaphragmatic position
   i. By suturing the oesophagus to the opposed right crus
   ii. By gastropexy
3. Construction of an acute angle between the abdominal oesophagus and the gastric fundus by:
   i. Suturing the fundus to the oesophagus
   ii. Suturing the fundus to the undersurface of the left diaphragm
   iii. Wrapping the fundus around and suturing it to the abdominal oesophagus (Nissen fundoplication)
4. Weakening of the oesophageal longitudinal muscle by:
   i. Circumferential oesophageal myotomy
   ii. Multiple, short, sector myotomies
5. Adequate gastric drainage if there is an element of duodenal stenosis
6. A lowering of any gastric hypersecretion by vagotomy

SPECIFIC SURGICAL PROCEDURES

1. Fundoplication
i.   Reduction of hernia at laparotomy
ii.   A wide bore stomach tube is passed into the oesophagus to prevent too tight a closure of right crus
iii. The margins of the right crus are defined and approximated behind the oesophagus
iv.   Mobilisation of the proximal stomach by division of gastro-splenic omentum
v.   The mobilised fundus is wrapped around and sutured in front of the abdominal oesophagus to produce an 'unspillable inkwell' effect
vi.   Vagotomy, pyloroplasty or Boerema gastropexy can be added

2. Belsey operation
i.   Thoracotomy through bed of 7th or 8th rib
ii.   The acute angle of entry of the oesophagus into the stomach, and a length of intra-abdominal oesophagus is produced by a series of mattress sutures which pass from the oesophagus (a few cm above OGJ); to the fundus (an equal distance from OGJ) to the diaphragm from below upwards; (2 cm from the hernial ring) then back through the diaphragm to pick up fundus and oesophagus again
iii. The right crus is then approximated behind the oesophagus

3. Collis operation
i.   Left thoraco-abdominal approach
ii.   Approximation of right crus *in front* of the oesophagus
iii. The fundus of the stomach is sutured to the undersurface of left dome of diaphragm to maintain an acute angle between the abdominal oesophagus and stomach

4. Gastropexy
i.   *Boerema anterior gastropexy:* Fixation of anterior surface of stomach (adjacent to lesser curve) to the linea alba
ii.   *Hill posterior gastropexy:* Fixation of lesser curve (and posterior phreno-oesophageal ligament) to median arcuate ligament

Advantages of gastropexv over conventional procedures:
i. Simple, rapid, safe
ii. Repair of hiatus is optional depending on condition of patient
iii. Published series report a lower radiological recurrence and higher symptomatic cure than conventional procedures
iv. The advantages of abdominal approach

ADVANTAGES OF ABDOMINAL OVER THORACIC REPAIR

1. Laparotomy is less painful
2. Laparotomy is safer in the middle-aged obese patient
3. A satisfactory examination of other intra-abdominal organs can be performed
4. Surgery can be performed to associated abnormalities (cholelithiasis and duodenal ulceration)

FURTHER READING

Boerema, I. (1969) Hiatus hernia: Repair by right-sided subhepatic, anterior gastropexy. *Surgery,* **65,** 884-893.

Davidson, J. S. (1972) Circumferential oesophageal myotomy. *British Journal of Surgery,* **59,** 938-947.

Franklin, R. H., Iweze, F.I., Owen-Smith, M.S. (1973) Fundoplication for hiatus hernia. *British Journal of Surgery,* **60,** 65-69.

Hill, L.D. (1967) An effective operation for hiatal hernia. *Annals of Surgery,* **166,** 681-692.

Leigh Collis, J. (1970) An appraisal of the methods for treating hiatus hernia and its complications. *Annals of the Royal College of Surgeons of England,* **46,** 338-349.

Mullard, K. S. (1972) The surgical treatment of diaphragmatic oesophageal hiatus hernia. *Annals of the Royal College of Surgeons of England,* **50,** 73-91.

Royston, C.M.S., Dowling, B.L., Spencer, J. (1975) Antrectomy with Roux-en-Y anastomosis in the treatment of peptic oesophagitis with stricture. *British Journal of Surgery,* **62,** 605-607.

Duodenal ulceration

The ideal elective operation for chronic duodenal ulceration should guarantee the following criteria:
1. The lowest operative mortality
2. The lowest incidence of recurrent ulceration
3. The lowest incidence of postgastric operation syndromes

A prospective controlled trial (Leeds/York Trial) compared the clinical results of truncal vagotomy with gastroenterostomy, truncal vagotomy with antrectomy, and subtotal gastrectomy
1. Although there were no immediate deaths following gastric resection (antrectomy or gastrectomy) it is accepted that gastric resection carries a mortality of 1 or 2%
2. Recurrent ulceration is more common after vagotomy with gastroenterostomy (7 to 10%) than after vagotomy with antrectomy or subtotal gastrectomy (2 to 6%)
3. Except for mild episodic diarrhoea following vagotomy, postgastric operation syndromes occurred with equal frequency
4. The three groups of patients showed no statistical difference in the quality of result as assessed by Visick grading

Goligher, J.C. *et al.* (1968) Five to eight-year results of Leeds/York controlled trial of elective surgery for duodenal ulcer. *British Medical Journal,* ii, 781-787.
Goligher, J.C. *et al.* (1968) Clinical comparison of vagotomy and pyloroplasty with other forms of elective surgery for duodenal ulcer. *British Medical Journal,* ii, 787-789.

The popularity of vagotomy is based on the low operative mortality (less than 0.5%). Gastric resection (antrectomy) is then reserved for the 8% of patients with recurrent ulceration. Techniques of vagotomy have been modified to lower the incidence of postvagotomy syndromes:

Postvagotomy diarrhoea

24% after truncal vagotomy and drainage
12% after selective vagotomy and drainage
2% after highly selective vagotomy (without drainage)
Postvagotomy diarrhoea is thought to be due to rapid,
unregulated gastric emptying and to small bowel denervation

Johnston, D. *et al.* (1972) Vagotomy without diarrhoea. *British Medical Journal,*
iii, 788-790.
Kennedy, T. *et al.* (1973) Selective or truncal vagotomy. *British Journal of
Surgery,* **60**, 944-948.
McKelvey, S.T.D. (1970) Gastric incontinence and post-vagotomy diarrhoea.
British Journal of Surgery, **57**, 741-747.

Postvagotomy dumping

Dumping is significantly less frequent after highly selective
vagotomy than following truncal or selective vagotomy with
pyloroplasty

Humphrey, C.S. *et al.* (1972) Incidence of dumping after truncal and selective
vagotomy with pyloroplasty and highly selective vagotomy without drainage
procedure. *British Medical Journal,* iii, 785-788.

HIGHLY SELECTIVE VAGOTOMY

(Proximal gastric vagotomy. Parietal cell vagotomy)
Denervation of the secretory cell mass only. Innervation of the
antropyloroduodenal segment is intact via the anterior and
posterior nerves of Latarget. This obviates the need for a
drainage procedure
Severity of postvagotomy syndromes can be reduced to a
minimum with highly selective vagotomy without any increased
incidence of recurrent ulceration

Kennedy, T. *et al.* (1975) Proximal gastric vagotomy: interim results of a
randomised controlled trial. *British Medical Journal,* ii, 301-303.

Localised avascular necrosis of lesser curve

1. A rare but definite complication of HSV
2. Usually occurs on the third to sixth postoperative day
3. The ischaemic ulceration is usually high on the lesser
   curve and the margins of the perforation show ischaemic
   changes on biopsy
4. Suture of the greater omentum over the bare area of
   lesser curve has been suggested to minimise the risk
5. (The lesser curve has a much poorer blood supply than
   the greater curve, anterior or posterior surfaces. The
   submucous plexus is usually absent on the lesser curve)

Halvorsen, J.F. *et al.* (1975) Localised avascular necrosis of lesser curve of
stomach complicating highly selective vagotomy. *British Medical Journal,* ii,
590-591.

Vagal reinnervation of the lesser curve?

About one half of the patients who are Hollander-negative in the early postoperative period become Hollander-positive by the end of one year. This is probably due to partial vagal reinnervation of the parietal cell mass. Reperitonealisation of the lesser curve has been suggested to prevent reinnervation of the lesser curve from the Nerves of Latarget.

Amdrup, E. & Kragelund, E. (1971) Evidence for partial vagal reinnervation of the stomach after highly selective vagotomy without a drainage procedure for duodenal ulcer in man. *Gut,* **12,** 866.

THE HISTAMINE H_2-RECEPTOR ANTAGONISTS

The antiallergic antihistamines do not block histamine induced cardiac acceleration and gastric secretion. The H_2-receptor mediates cardiac acceleration and gastric secretion and is blocked by the new antihistamines, burinamide, metiamide and cimetidine.

Gastric secretion induced by vagal stimulation, histamine and pentagastrin is inhibited.

Metiamide

1. Has been shown to inhibit nocturnal acid secretion in patients with duodenal ulceration
2. Produces significant reduction in night pain and total antacid consumption. Daytime pain is diminished
3. The healing of duodenal ulcers, assessed by serial endoscopy, is significantly increased in patients receiving metiamide
4. Reversible granulocytopenia has occurred six times during the administration of metiamide. (Possibly related to its thiourea structure)

Cimetidine

1. A non-thiourea H_2-receptor antagonist
2. Less toxic in dogs than metiamide
3. May be more active than metiamide
4. Therapeutic value being investigated

Blackwood, W.S. *et al.,* (1976) Cimetidine in duodenal ulcer. *Lancet,* ii, 174-176.

Lancet (1975) Treatment of duodenal ulcer by metiamide. A Multicentre Trial. *Lancet,* ii, 779-781.

Milton-Thompson, G.J. *et al.* (1974) Inhibition of nocturnal acid secretion in duodenal ulcer by one oral dose of metiamide. *Lancet,* i, 693-694.

Pounder, R.E. *et al.* (1975) Relief of duodenal ulcer symptoms by oral metiamide. *British Medical Journal,* ii, 307-309.

Complications of gastrectomy

1. HAEMORRHAGE
  i. **Intraperitoneal**
     a. Torn splenic capsule
     b. Bleeding from an insecurely ligated major vascular pedicle or omental vessel
  ii. **Intraluminal**
     a. Suture line haemorrhage. If severe, controlled by gastrotomy in the gastric remnant and over-sewing of the suture line
     b. Bleeding from an ulcer in the gastric remnant not observed at operation
     c. Bleeding diathesis

2. ACUTE GASTRIC (REMNANT) DILATION
  i. Risk of suture line disruption
  ii. Significant fluid and electrolyte loss into the gastric remnant
  iii. Prevented by nasogastric decompression of the gastric remnant until the ileus has resolved

3 PANCREATITIS
  i. Rare, but post-operative pancreatitis has a mortality of 50%
  ii. May be related to pancreatic trauma during mobilisation of a posterior penetrating duodenal or gastric ulcer
  iii. Post-gastrectomy pancreatitis may occur without apparent pancreatic trauma
  iv. The Duct of Santorini may be damaged during mobilisation of the duodenal bulb and discharge pancreatic secretions into the peritoneal cavity

See Acute pancreatitis p. 29

4. DUODENAL STUMP LEAKAGE
The commonest cause of mortality in gastric resection
Usually occurs in the 4th or 5th postoperative day
Predisposing factors
  i. Extensive mobilisation of the duodenal bulb resulting in duodenal ischaemia
  ii. Difficult closure of the duodenal stump especially if a large oedematous ulcer is penetrating the head of the pancreas
  iii. Afferent loop obstruction

Treatment
  i.   Immediate and adequate drainage of bile and pancreatic fluid preferably by sump drainage to protect the skin
  ii. Maintenance of fluid and electrolyte balance
  iii. Spontaneous closure can be expected if the afferent loop is not obstructed

5. AFFERENT LOOP OBSTRUCTION

Aetiology
  i.   Stomal oedema in the immediate postoperative period
  ii.   Narrowing or stenosis of the afferent loop by sutures during construction of the gastrojejunostomy stoma
  iii. Kinking of a long afferent loop
  iv.   Distortion of the gastrojejunostomy by active or healing stomal ulcer

Presentation
  i.   Duodenal stump leakage early postoperatively
  ii.   Intermittent epigastric pain and distension relieved suddenly and often synchronously with bile-stained vomiting
  iii. Malabsorption
  iv.   As a late acute illness with pain, distension, dehydration and the danger of ischaemic necrosis of an enormously dilated afferent loop

Treatment
  i.   Revision gastrectomy to provide an adequate stoma with shortening of the afferent loop if necessary
  ii.   Entero-enterostomy between the afferent and efferent loops

6. EFFERENT LOOP OBSTRUCTION

  i.   For several days postoperatively oedema at the stoma can delay gastric emptying causing excessive nasogastric aspirates
  ii.   Following retro-colic Polya gastrectomy, small bowel can pass through the defect in the transverse mesocolon Prevented by closing this defect and suturing the 'window' in the mesocolon to the gastric remnant so that the anastomosis lies wholly in the infracolic compartment.
  iii. Following ante-colic Polya gastrectomy a loop of small bowel (Stammers loop) can pass between the gastrojejunostomy anastomosis anteriorly and the transverse colon posteriorly, causing intestinal obstruction

7. ANASTOMOTIC LEAK

Aetiology
i.   Ischaemia. The gastric remnant can be rendered ischaemic if the left gastric artery is ligated at its origin and subsequently during the procedure a splenectomy becomes necessary
ii. Gastric (remnant) dilation
iii. Technical imperfections
iv. Cachexia, hypoproteinaemia, etc.

Treatment
i.   Immediate and adequate drainage with closure of dehiscence where possible. (Rarely will an ischaemic gastric remnant require excision and restoration of continuity by a Roux loop of jejunum.) A nasogastric tube should be passed well into the efferent loop to allow feeding
ii. Maintenance of fluid and electrolyte balance while awaiting spontaneous closure of gastric fistula

8. SUBPHRENIC ABSCESS

Aetiology
i.   Duodenal stump leakage
ii. Anastomotic leak
iii. Intraperitoneal haemorrhage
iv. Splenectomy

9. STOMAL ULCERATION

Usually occurs at the origin of the efferent loop of a Polya gastrectomy. May present with pain, perforation, haemorrhage, gastrojejunocolic fistula, or obstruction at the gastrojejunal anastomosis

Treatment
i.   Uncomplicated stomal ulceration can be treated by supradiaphragmatic truncal vagotomy (left thoracotomy). This does not permit inspection of the gastrojejunal anastomosis
ii. Stomal ulcers should be assessed by laparotomy
  a. Distortion and stenosis of the gastrojejunal anastomosis will require revision gastrectomy. The stomal ulcer is resected with the gastrectomy specimen and the gastrojejunal anastomosis reconstructed. The jejunojejunal anastomosis (the original juxtagastric ends of the afferent and efferent loop) will be sited either on the new afferent or efferent loop depending on the length of the original afferent loop

b. An uncomplicated ulcer is treated by selective vagotomy

c. A perforated stomal ulcer without anastomotic stenosis can be treated by closure of the perforation and selective vagotomy

d. Bleeding from a stomal ulcer can be treated by gastrojejunotomy, under-running of the ulcer and selective vagotomy

e. A gastrojejunocolic fistula is resected with the gastrectomy specimen and the gastrojejunostomy reconstructed. It is safer for both ends of the colon to be brought to the surface and for colonic continuity to be restored as a secondary procedure

Crohn's disease

Crohn's disease is a granulomatous disease of unknown aetiology. The whole thickness of bowel wall is infiltrated by lymphocytes, plasma cells and non-caseating tubercles. The submucosa especially is thickened. The mucosa is usually spared. Crypt abscesses open on to the mucosa but may discharge to the serosal surface forming a fistula either with skin, bladder, vagina or gut.

In one large series:
   60% had small bowel involvement only
   17% had small and large bowel involvement
   17% had large bowel involvement only
   A small percentage will have involvement of mouth, pharynx, oesophagus or stomach

A bimodal age incidence has been demonstrated:
   Young adults, and at around seventy years
   Terminal ileal disease tends to affect young patients
   Recto-sigmoid and perianal disease commoner in the elderly
   Colonic Crohn's diffusely scattered through all age groups

NUTRITIONAL ASPECTS OF CROHN'S DISEASE

1. Weight loss and hypoproteinaemia
   i.   Anorexia
   ii. Loss of absorbing surface: Inflammation
                                    Fistulae
                                    Surgical resection or bypass
   iii. Loss of blood, plasma protein, fluid and electrolytes from inflamed bowel. (Protein losing enteropathy)

2. Anaemia
   i.   Iron deficiency: chronic blood loss
   ii. B^{12} deficiency: diseased or resected terminal ileum
   iii. Folate deficiency: malabsorption and increased requirement
   iv. Toxic marrow depression

MEDICAL TREATMENT OF CROHN'S DISEASE

1. Salazopyrine
2. Steroids
3. Azathioprine
   Indications:
   i. Active disease not responding to steroids alone and where surgery is contra-indicated
   ii. Fistulae—some will improve or heal
   iii. Per-operatively to reduce suture line recurrence, dehiscence and fistula formation
4. Correction of anaemia
5. Correction of hypoproteinaemia
   i. Will improve as inflammation is suppressed
   ii. Parenteral alimentation may be necessary, especially as a prelude to surgery
6. Control of diarrhoea
   i. Low fat diet if steatorrhoea is a feature
   ii. Codeine. Lomotil
   iii. Cholestyramine. Bile salts not absorbed by ileum have cathartic action on colon

INDICATIONS FOR SURGERY

1. Abscess
2. Fistulae
3. Stricture
4. Perforation
5. Obstruction
6. Failure to suppress active disease by medical means where the disease is not so extensive that surgery is contra-indicated, and where an operative mortality of approximately 3% is acceptable
7. Uveitis, recurrent polyarthritis, pyoderma gangrenosa

SURGICAL MANAGEMENT OF CROHN'S DISEASE

1. Drainage of abscess
   i. Abdominal wall or perianal. Invariably results in a fistula

2.   Excisional surgery

Should only be performed when general health is good. A compromise should be sought between adequate clearance of diseased bowel and removing only sufficient normal bowel to allow safe anastomosis

   i.   Resection of localised small bowel disease with restoration of continuity

   ii.   Limited right hemicolectomy for terminal ileal disease anastomosing ileum to ascending colon

   iii. With normal ileum and extensive colonic disease proctocolectomy and ileostomy is indicated. Even if the rectum is histologically normal, ileo-rectal anastomosis is unsatisfactory in terms of operative mortality and recurrence

   iv.   In the few patients with localised recto-sigmoid and severe perianal disease, excisional surgery with terminal colostomy is satisfactory

3.   Surgery designed to defunction diseased bowel

Where it is safer to perform bypass or defunctioning surgery than excisional surgery. Indications defined by poor general condition of patient and severity of local disease, e.g. fistula or abscess. Usually a preliminary to subsequent resection

   i.   End-to-side ileotransverse colostomy in severe disease of terminal ileum

   ii.   Defunctioning ileostomy in patients with extensive colo-rectal involvement

   iii. Rarely a loop colostomy in patients with recto-sigmoid or perianal disease. (Usually primary excisional surgery is possible)

FURTHER READING
British Journal of Surgery (1972) Symposium on Crohn's Disease. *British Journal of Surgery,* **59**, 806-829.
British Medical Journal (1975) Sulphasalazine for Crohn's Disease? *British Medical Journal,* ii, 297-298.

Ulcerative colitis

PATHOLOGY

Mild:　Submucosal chronic inflammatory cells
Atrophy of mucosa
Decreased number of goblet cells in crypts of
Lieberkuhn

Severe:　Polymorphs in lamina propria
Pronounced loss of goblet cells
Decreased number of crypts of Lieberkuhn
Crypt abscesses
Ulceration and granulation

COMPLICATIONS

Local:　Blood loss. Anaemia
Protein loss
Acute toxic dilation of colon
Perforation
Stricture
Carcinoma

General:　Large joint arthropathy
Uveitis
Spondylitis
Erythema nodosum
Pyoderma gangrenosa

MEDICAL MANAGEMENT OF ACUTE ULCERATIVE COLITIS

A suggested 5 day intensive i.v. regimen
1. Water only by mouth
2. i.v. replacement of fluid and electrolytes
3. Parenteral feeding (50 to 60 kcals/Kg)
4. i.v. Prednisone, 60 mg/day
5. Blood transfusion to maintain haemoglobin
6. Twice daily steroid retention enemas
(No antibiotics—risk of enterocolitis)

INDICATIONS FOR SURGERY

In acute attack
Failure to respond to medical treatment
Acute toxic dilation
Perforation

In chronic disease
    Continuous, disabling symptoms
    Recurrent polyarthritis
    Fibrous stricture
    Carcinoma or the risk of developing carcinoma

SURGICAL TREATMENT

In acute attack
  i.   Transverse colostomy. In fulminating cases where the patient is too ill for colectomy. See references for further discussion
  ii. Colectomy, ileostomy, and recto-sigmoid mucous fistula:
      a.   With secondary excision of rectum when the patient's condition permits
      b.   With later conversion to ileo-rectal anastomosis
  iii. Panproctocolectomy with ileostomy

In chronic attack
  i.   Colectomy with ileo-rectal anastomosis with or without a temporary ileostomy
  ii. Subtotal colectomy with caecoproctostomy
  iii. Panproctocolectomy and ileostomy

COMPLICATIONS OF SURGERY

General: Haemorrhage
            Pulmonary infection and collapse
            Wound sepsis
            DVT, pulmonary embolism
Specific: Peritonitis. Localised abscess
                         Septicaemic shock
            Adhesions to bare colonic bed
            Adhesions to pelvic floor
            Internal hernia through para-ileostomy space
            Ileostomy prolapse, regression or stenosis
            Perineal sinus
            Skin excoriation related to ileostomy
            Para-ileostomy hernia
            Retraction of recto-sigmoid mucous fistula

PATIENTS WITH ULCERATIVE COLITIS AT RISK OF DEVELOPING CARCINOMA

    Clinically severe first attack
    Panproctocolitis
    Chronic continuous symptoms (rather than intermittent attacks)
    Where the onset of colitis was in childhood or early adult life

The clinical diagnosis of carcinoma complicating ulcerative colitis is difficult because the symptoms of carcinoma may be confused with an exacerbation of ulcerative colitis

The radiological recognition of early carcinoma can be difficult in an already diseased colon. The following methods have been advocated to detect malignant change:

1.   Serial rectal biopsies to detect in-situ mucosal changes

Evans, D.J. & Pollock, D.J. (1972) In-situ and invasive carcinoma of the colon in patients with ulcerative colitis. *Gut,* **13**, 566-570.

Morson, B.C. & Pang, L.S.C. (1967) Rectal biopsy as an aid to cancer control in ulcerative colitis. *Gut,* **8**, 423-434

2.   Serial estimations of carcinoembryonic antigen in serum and faeces. The usefulness of this test may not live up to expectation

Dilawari, J.B. *et al.* (1975) Estimation of carcinoembryonic antigen in ulcerative colitis with special reference to malignant change. *Gut,* **16**, 255-260.

FURTHER READING

Aylett, S.O. (1970) The fulminating case of ulcerative colitis or Crohn's Disease. *Proceedings of the Royal Society of Medicine,* **63**, Suppl., 75-76.

Aylett, S.O. (1971) Ileorectal anastomosis: Review 1952-1968. *Proceedings of the Royal Society of Medicine,* **64**, 967-971.

Goligher, J.C. & Lintott, D. (1975) Experience with 26 reservoir ileostomies. *British Journal of Surgery,* **62**,   893-900.

Lee, E.C.G. & Dowling, B.L. (1972) Perimuscular excision of the rectum for Crohn's disease and ulcerative colitis. *British Journal of Surgery,* **59**, 29-32.

Truelove, S.C. & Jewell, D.P. (1974) Intensive intravenous regimen for severe attacks of ulcerative colitis. *Lancet,* i, 1067-1070.

Weakley, F.L. & Turnbull, R.B. (1970) Exclusion and decompression for toxic dilation of the colon in ulcerative colitis. *Proceedings of the Royal Society of Medicine,* **63**, Suppl., 73-75.

Webster, G.U. & Howard, R.R.S. (1973) Subtotal colectomy and caecoproctostomy. *British Journal of Surgery,* **60**, 42-44.

Diverticular disease of colon

PATHOGENESIS

Low fibre diet

$\downarrow$

Inappropriate segmentation of colonic circular muscle

$\downarrow$

'segmental intraluminal hypertension'

$\downarrow$

Gross thickening of circular muscle
Pulsion diverticulae

TREATMENT OF UNCOMPLICATED DIVERTICULAR DISEASE

High residue diet: Fresh fruit and vegetables
Wholemeal bread and flour
Unprocessed bran
Bulk purgatives
Antispasmodics

Intraluminal colonic pressure is abnormally high in diverticular disease, and gastro-intestinal transit time is prolonged

Unprocessed bran lowers intraluminal pressure and shortens transit time

Findlay J. M. *et al.* (1974) Effects of unprocessed bran on colon function in normal subjects and in diverticular disease. *Lancet,* **1**, 146-149.

COMPLICATIONS OF DIVERTICULAR DISEASE

1. Diverticulitis: Localised peritonitis
   Generalised peritonitis
2. Haemorrhage
3. Colonic stenosis and obstruction
4. Fistula formation: Vesicocolic
   Enterocolic
   Colo-colic
   Colo-vaginal
5. Small bowel intestinal obstruction

INDICATIONS FOR SURGERY
1. Severe progressive inflammatory disease. (Recurrent episodes of acute diverticulitis)
2. Failure to control long standing symptoms by medical means.
3. Colonic stricture and the possibility of malignancy
4. General peritonitis
5. Massive, continuous, uncontrolled haemorrhage
6. Fistulae

TREATMENT OF COMPLICATIONS OF DIVERTICULAR DISEASE

1. Acute diverticulitis with localised peritonitis
Intravenous fluids
Antibiotics

2. Acute diverticulitis with generalised peritonitis
Intensive treatment of fluid depletion and shock (hypovolaemic or bacteraemic) in preparation for surgery
   i.   Purulent turbid peritonitis (Rupture of pericolic abscess)
        a. Peritoneal toilet
        b. Pelvic drain
        c. Antibiotics
        d. Management of ileus
   ii. Faecal peritonitis
        a. Resection of inflamed bowel without primary anastomosis:
            Mikulicz resection
            Hartmann resection
            Restoration of colonic continuity at a secondary procedure
        b. Defunctioning colostomy and pelvic drainage.
            An alternative if resection is not technically possible

3. Massive, continuous, uncontrolled haemorrhage
In many series reviewing haemorrhage in diverticular disease, the source of the bleeding in more than half the cases occurred in the ascending or proximal transverse colon
   i.   Total colectomy with ileostomy or ileorectal anastomosis
   ii. Subtotal colectomy with caecoproctostomy
   iii. Conservative resection following accurate localisation of bleeding site by selective arteriography

Eisenberg, H, Laufer, I, Skillman, J.J. (1973) Arteriographic diagnosis and management of suspected colonic diverticular haemorrhage. *Gastroenterology*, **64**, 1091-1100.

4.   Fistulae

Initial defunctioning colostomy to allow inflammation at the site of the fistula to settle

At a secondary procedure:

i.   Excision of diseased colon and fistulous tract with colonic anastomosis

ii.   Layered closure of the organ involved by the fistula (bladder, vagina, etc.)

iii.   Interposition of omentum

Closure of colostomy

FURTHER READING

Bolt, D.E. (1973) Diverticular disease of the large intestine. *Annals of the Royal College of Surgeons of England,* **53**, 237-245.

Burkitt, D.P., Walker, A.R.P. & Painter, N.S. (1972) Effect of dietary fibre on stools and transit-times and its role in the causation of disease. *Lancet,* ii, 1408-1411.

Painter, N.S., Almeida, A.Z. & Colebourne, K.W. (1972) Unprocessed bran in treatment of diverticular disease of the colon. *British Medical Journal,* ii, 137-140.

Penfold, J.C.B. (1973) Management of uncomplicated diverticular disease by colonic resection in patients at St. Mark's Hospital, 1964-9. *British Journal of Surgery,* **60**, 695-698.

Reilly, M.C.T. (1970) Colonic diverticula: Surgical management. *British Medical Journal,* iii, 570-573.

Tagart, R.E.B. (1974) General peritonitis and haemorrhage complicating colonic diverticular disease. *Annals of the Royal College of Surgeons of England,* **55**, 175-183.

Acute pancreatitis

Haemorrhagic necrotising pancreatitis has a mortality of 20 to 25%. Death is caused by:
1. Shock
2. Acute renal failure
3. Retroperitoneal abscess formation
4. Gastrointestinal haemorrhage

(Clinically and prognostically different to recurrent acute pancreatitis which is a mild disease with a mortality of less than 1%)

CLINICAL AND LABORATORY CRITERIA

Pain, vomiting, paralytic ileus
Severe pancreatitis associated with:
    Shock
    Cardiorespiratory failure
    Acute renal failure
    Prolonged paralytic ileus
    Disseminated intravascular coagulation (DIC)
    Serum calcium lower than 1.9mmol/l (7.6mg/100ml)
    Methaemalbumin positive
94% of patients with acute pancreatitis have serum amylase
    above 1,000 Somogyi units (1875 IU/l)
Such elevated levels not usually associated with:
    Perforated duodenal ulcer
    Mesenteric vascular occlusion
    Duodenal stump 'blow-out'
Degree of elevation of amylase not proportional to severity of
    illness

ASSOCIATED AETIOLOGICAL FACTORS

1. Biliary disease (40 to 60%)
The theory of reflux of altered or infected bile into pancreatic duct. Biliary pathogens deconjugate bilirubin. Unconjugated bile known to damage acinar cells.
2. Alcohol (up to 25%)
Possibly by stimulating pancreatic exocrine secretion while causing spasm of sphincter of Oddi or by toxic metabolic effect on acinar cells

3.   A previous Polya gastrectomy

The theory of reflux of activated pancreatic proteolytic enzymes from duodenum into pancreatic duct. Associated with Polya and not Bilroth I gastrectomy. Lack of free drainage from the afferent loop is probably important

4.   Postoperative

Usually following procedures for peptic ulceration or biliary stones. Associated with a very high mortality

5.   Open and closed abdominal trauma
6.   Steroid therapy
7.   Hyperparathyroidism
8.   Endoscopic retrograde cholangiopancreatography(ERCP)
9.   Pregnancy. Invariably runs a benign course

TREATMENT

1.   Shock

Blood and plasma expanders under CVP control to replace huge deficit of plasma volume. Shock may be irreversible due to the presence of vaso-active substances

2.   Trasylol (Aprotinin)

Proven by controlled trial to be of therapeutic value

Trypsin and Kallikrein Inhibitor. Inhibits vaso-active enzymes

200,000u stat. 200,000u 6 hrly i.v. for 5 days

Trasylol reduces death rate significantly and reduces severity of illness

3.   Supression of pancreatic exocrine secretion
   i.   Nasogastric suction
   ii.   Anticholinergics (of unproven value)
   iii. Glucagon
      1 mg. i.v. stat
      Infusion 1-1.5mg. 4 hrly for 24-96 h
      Known to decrease pancreatic exocrine secretion
      Rapid relief of pain
      Produces clinical improvement
      Decreases plasma amylase
      Lowers serum calcium further by releasing calcitonin
      Results of Glucagon encouraging. Value not yet proven
      by controlled trial

4.   Antibiotics

Of unproven value in preventing abscess formation

5.   Renal failure

Diagnosed by a blood urea of over 16.6mmol/l (100mg/100ml) after restoring circulating volume

Early peritoneal dialysis

Caused by acute tubular necrosis or DIC affecting glomerular tuft

6. Peritoneal lavage

Claimed that peritoneal lavage has a therapeutic value by removing proteolytic enzymes from peritoneal cavity.

Trasylol can be instilled

Performed via catheter inserted percutaneously or at laparotomy

7. Cardiorespiratory failure

Pulmonary congestion, atelectasis and pleural effusions (Suggested that surfactant is de-natured)

Treat a falling Po_2 by 100% oxygen

Treat respiratory failure by positive pressure respiration

Digoxin and diuretics if required

8. Hypocalcaemia

Monitor serum calcium especially if Glucagon therapy in progress

10% calcium gluconate i.v. repeated as necessary

9. Laparotomy

Should be performed early if diagnostic uncertainty exists

Some authorities believe that all severe cases should undergo laparotomy, aspiration of necrotic retroperitoneal mass, and drainage

In the presence of an infected or obstructed biliary tree, cholecystostomy, T-tube drainage of CBD or sphincteroplasty may be performed

COMPLICATIONS AND THEIR MANAGEMENT

1. Abscess
   i. The commonest and most serious late complication
   ii. Presents with mass, swinging fever, clinical deterioration
   iii. Usually presents during third or fourth week
   iv. Abscess often multilocular with retroperitoneal, perinephric and subphrenic components
   v. Drainage does not predispose to fistula formation
2. Pseudocysts
   i. Peak incidence at 3 weeks
   ii. Presence of a cyst not in itself an indication for drainage
   iii. Pancreatic cysts can resolve. Treat if cyst is enlarging or leaking
   iv. Cysts appearing early have friable, inflamed walls and only external drainage is possible
   v. Established cysts are best treated by cystogastrotomy or by cysto-jejunostomy-en-Roux

3. Gastrointestinal haemorrhage
    i.   Usually a terminal event
    ii.   Usually due to acute gastric erosions
    iii. Gastric perforation can occur
    iv.   Associated with extensive pancreatic necrosis and abscess formation
    v.   Surgery is rarely of benefit
4. Duodenal ileus
    i.   Suggests continuing pancreatic inflammation or abscess formation
    ii.   Treat by prolonged i.v. fluids and nasogastric suction
    iii. Feeding jejunostomy or gastro-enterostomy may be necessary
    iv.   Exclude retroperitoneal, perinephric or subphrenic abscess
5. Burst abdomen
6. Recurrent attacks
7. Diabetes
8. Colonic and duodenal necrosis
9. Wound dehiscence

FURTHER READING

Condon, J.R., Knight, M. & Day, J.L. (1973) Glucagon therapy in acute pancreatitis. *British Journal of Surgery,* **60,** 509-511.

Trapnell, J.E. (1971) Management of the complications of acute pancreatitis. *Annals of the Royal College of Surgeons of England,* **49,** 361-372.

Trapnell, J.E. (1974) Acute pancreatitis. *British Journal of Hospital Medicine,* **12,** 193-203.

Trapnell, J.E., Rigby, C.C., Talbot, C.H. & Duncan, E.H.L. (1974) A controlled trial of Trasylol in the treatment of acute pancreatitis. *British Journal of Surgery,* **61,** 177-182.

Portal hypertension

Ideally, bleeding from oesophageal and gastric varices should be stopped by conservative means, and treatment directed over weeks or months to reverse any hepatic decompensation. When hepatic function is maximally improved and in the absence of specific contra-indication, a portal systemic decompression should be performed.

DIAGNOSIS

The stigmata of cirrhosis, hepatic failure and encephalopathy should be sought. The diagnosis of portal hypertension is questionable in the absence of splenomegaly but the size of the spleen is not proportional to the degree of portal hypertension. Since patients with cirrhosis may bleed from other sites (e.g. gastric erosions, duodenal ulceration) the bleeding site should be confirmed by fiberoptic oesophagoscopy. In the presence of recent evidence of variceal bleeding (e.g. thrombus adherent to oesophageal mucosa) the instrument should not be passed beyond.

CLASSIFICATION OF PORTAL HYPERTENSION

1. **Pre-hepatic portal hypertension**
   Portal vein thrombosis is associated with:
   i. Neonatal umbilical sepsis
   ii. Exchange transfusion
   iii. Suppurative pyelephlebitis complicating acute appendicitis
   iv. Acute and chronic osteomyelitis
   v. A thrombosed portacaval shunt

2. **Hepatic portal hypertension**
   Commonest causes of cirrhosis are:
   i. Cryptogenic
   ii. Chronic active hepatitis
   iii. Chronic progressive hepatitis
   iv. Alcoholic cirrhosis
   v. Primary biliary cirrhosis
   vi. Haemochromatosis
   vii. Wilson's disease (hepato-lenticular degeneration)

Except for chronic active hepatitis and Wilson's disease, (which present in the 2nd decade) the other causes of cirrhosis present most commonly in 5th to 7th decades

3. **Post-hepatic portal hypertension**
    Obstruction to hepatic veins caused by:
    i.   Constrictive pericarditis
    ii. Budd-Chiari Syndrome (hepatic vein occlusion)
        a. Spread of renal carcinoma along the inferior vena cava
        b. Polycythaemia rubra vera
        c. Oral contraceptives
        d. Thrombophlebitis migrans
    iii. Jamaican veno-occlusive disease (Bush Tea)

IN MOST SERIES OF VARICEAL BLEEDING

60% — Bleeding stopped by conservative means
25% — Recurrent haemorrhage. Emergency surgery must be
      considered
15% — Uncontrolled haemorrhage is a terminal event in
      advanced hepatic failure

Prognosis in emergency and elective surgery is closely related to hepatic function. In pre-hepatic portal hypertension, where liver function is usually normal, operative morbidity and mortality is at its lowest

1. **Criteria for a favourable prognosis**
    i.   Bilirubin—less than 25μmol/l (1.5mg/100ml)
    ii. Albumin—greater than 30g/l (3g/100ml)
    iii. No ascites
    iv. No encephalopathy
    v.   Good nutrition
2. **Criteria for an unfavourable prognosis**
    i.   Bilirubin—greater than 50μmol/l (3mg/100ml)
    ii. Albumin—less than 20g/l (2g/100ml)
    iii. Poorly controlled ascites
    iv. The presence of encephalopathy
    v.   Poor state of nutrition

(In alcoholic cirrhosis especially, abstention and medical treatment can result in marked improvement in liver function, and therefore prognostic criteria)

CONSERVATIVE MANAGEMENT OF VARICEAL BLEEDING

1. Replacement of blood lost with fresh blood
2. Vitamin K
3. Measures to prevent hepatic pre-coma:
    i.   Colonic washout
    ii. Oral non-absorbable antibiotics
4. Vasopressin 20u in 200 ml. 5% Dextrose i.v.
5. Sengstaken—Blakemore tube for 24 to 48 hours

EMERGENCY SURGERY TO STOP VARICEAL BLEEDING

(In this desperate situation operative mortality approaches 50%)
1. **Surgery directly to the varices**
   i. Transthoracic, transoesophageal ligation of varices(Boerema—Crile Operation)
      a. Approached through bed of 8th rib
      b. Arterial clamp applied to lower isolated oesophagus to prevent undue bleeding
      c. Longitudinal oesophagotomy
      d. Under-running of columns of varices by continuous suture
   ii. Transthoracic, oesophageal transection (mucosal or complete) (Milnes—Walker Operation)
      a. Longitudinal oesophageal myotomy
      b. Mucosa dissected out as a tube
      c. Mucosa transected, varices ligated, and mucosa reanastomosed
   iii. Subcardiac porto-azygous disconnection (Tanner Operation)
      a. Division of vessels entering greater and lesser curves of body and fundus of stomach
      b. Proximal gastric transection and reanastomosis

Advantages
   i. Portal blood flow is not diverted away from the liver and therefore liver function is not adversely affected (Hepatic failure is a common complication of portal systemic decompression—PSD)
   ii. Haemorrhage is controlled early in the operation

Disadvantages
   i. Anastomotic breakdown is a major cause of death in these patients with poor healing potential. (Mucosal oesophageal transection minimises this complication)
   ii. Portal hypertension is not lowered and unless contra-indicated, a second operation for PSD will be necessary
   iii. Transthoracic procedures may not stop bleeding from gastric varices

2. **Surgery to lower portal hypertension**
   i. Emergency portacaval shunt
      Has an unacceptable mortality in the emergency situation
   ii. Mesenterico-caval anastomosis (jump graft)
      Side-to-side Dacron graft between superior mesenteric vein and inferior vena cava
      Claimed to have an acceptable mortality in the favourable prognostic group and the necessity for two major surgical procedures is avoided

ELECTIVE SURGERY TO LOWER PORTAL HYPERTENSION

Portal systemic decompression is contra-indicated in the presence of encephalopathy

Over the age of 60 years encephalopathy as a complication of PSD increases rapidly

PSD affords maximal protection against further variceal bleeding.

1. **Portocaval shunt**
   i. A patent portal vein must be confirmed by portal venography
   ii. An end-to-side anastomosis is usually performed
   iii. A side-to-side anastomosis is technically much more difficult and offers no definite advantages
   iv. Usually performed through a long right subcostal incision
   v. 10% operative mortality
   vi. 3% shunt thrombosis
   vii. 20% of patients will develop encephalopathy

2. **Lieno-renal shunt**
   i. 10% operative mortality
   ii. 20% shunt thrombosis
   iii. 10% of patients will develop encephalopathy
   iv. The incidence of shunt patency is proportional to the diameter of the splenic vein. Therefore this operation is often unsuitable for children

3. **Mesenterico-caval shunt (jump graft)**
   i. May be the only method of PSD available when portal vein is thrombosed, or when a previous portacaval shunt has thrombosed
   ii. Has an excellent record of graft patency
   iii. Claimed not to produce encephalopathy because shunt is peripheral and because continued portal blood flow to the liver helps to preserve residual hepatic function
   iv. Alternatively, if at any time the haemodynamic situation requires it, hepatopetal blood flow is still possible.

4. **Warren's operation**
   i. Distal spleno-renal shunt and gastrosplenic isolation with spleen *in situ*
   ii. An attempt at selective decompression of gastro-oesophageal varices without disturbing the superior and inferior mesenteric veins or portal vein
   iii. Theoretically this should provide the least opportunity for encephalopathy to develop while maintaining portal blood flow and therefore, an undisturbed hepatic function

FURTHER READING

Johnston, G.W. & Rodgers, R.W. (1973) A review of 15 years' experience in the use of sclerotherapy in the control of acute haemorrhage from oesophageal varices. *British Journal of Surgery,* **60**, 797-800

Kirby, R., Burke, F.D. & Jones, J.D.T. (1975) Emergency and elective surgical treatment of portal hypertension. *Annals of the Royal College of Surgeons of England,* **57**, 148-158.

Marks, C. (1976) The anatomical basis for portal decompressive surgery. *Annals of the Royal College of Surgeons of England,* **58**, 293-299.

Pugh, R.N.H., Murray-Lyon, I.M., Dawson, J.L., Pietroni, M.C. & Williams, R. (1973) Transection of the oesophagus for bleeding oesophageal varices. *British Journal of Surgery,* **60**, 646-649.

Rothwell-Jackson, R.L. & Hunt, A.H. (1971) The results obtained with emergency surgery in the treatment of persistent haemorrhage from gastro-oesophageal varices in the cirrhotic patient. *British Journal of Surgery,* **58**, 205-215.

Smith, M., Tuft, R.J., Davidson, A.R., Laws, J.W., Dawson, J.L. & Williams, R. (1974) Mesentericocaval 'jump' graft in management of portal hypertension: experience with 24 cases. *British Medical Journal,* iii, 705-708.

Waldran, R., Davis, M., Nunnerley, H. & Williams, R. (1974) Emergency endoscopy after gastrointestinal haemorrhage in 50 patients with portal hypertension. *British Medical Journal,* iv, 94-96.

Warren, W.D., Zeppa, R. & Fomon, J.J. (1967) Selective trans-splenic decompression of gastro-oesophageal varices by distal splenorenal shunt. *Annals of Surgery,* **166**, 437-455.

Gram-negative septicaemia and shock

Gradually during the antibiotic era, gram-negative organisms have become predominant in septicaemia

Endotoxaemia rather than bacteraemia is assumed to cause septic shock, which carries a mortality of 80%

Transient bacteraemia, invariably of no consequence, is common even in minor surgical procedures such as bladder catheterisation, sigmoidoscopy and biopsy, percutaneous liver biopsy and even barium enema examination

PATHOPHYSIOLOGY

1. Endotoxin (a complex lipopolysaccharide bound to cell wall protein) is produced from the cell wall of dead microorganisms
2. Endotoxin causes the release of chemical mediators such as kinins, serotonin, histamine, adrenaline and noradrenaline which produce intense vasospasm of arterioles and venules with pooling of blood in the microcirculation
3. Inadequate perfusion of vital organs with oxygenated blood causes:
   i. Anaerobic cellular metabolism
   ii. Increasing blood lactate and metabolic acidosis
   iii. Decrease of tissue stores of ATP
4. Lack of cellular energy (ATP) results in:
   i. Failure of sodium-potassium pump, loss of intracellular potassium and hyperkalaemia
   ii. Lysozomal release of enzymes (proteases, esterases, phosphatase) with cellular autodigestion
5. Capillary permeability is altered promoting the transfer of fluid from the intravascular to interstitial compartments
6. Endotoxin activation of coagulation system with disseminated intravascular coagulation (DIC)
   i. Fragmented RBC and thrombocytopenia on blood film
   ii. Hypofibrinogenaemia and consumption of other coagulation factors
   iii. Fibrinogen degradation products (FDP) in blood and urine

AETIOLOGY OF SEPTIC SHOCK

1. Most frequently occurs in the first (premature and newborn infants), seventh and eighth decades, in poor risk patients
2. Is most commonly seen as an infective complication of major surgery.The organism is often acquired from the hospital reservoir of resistant organisms (misuse and overuse of antibiotics)
3. Following manipulation or instrumentation in the presence of obstruction to, or bacterial overgrowth of:
   i. Urinary tract
   ii. Gastrointestinal tract
   iii. Biliary tree
   iv. Genital tract
   v. Skin (burns)
4. The following factors place the patient at greater risk:
   i. Diabetes mellitus, chronic uraemia, cirrhosis
   ii. Leukaemias, reticuloses, other malignancies
   iii. Steroids, immunosuppression, or antimitotic agents

BACTERIOLOGY (in order of frequency)

1. *Escherichia coli*
2. *Proteus species*
3. *Pseudomonas aeruginosa*
4. *Klebsiella*
5. *Enterobacter*
6. *Bacteroides fragilis*
   i. Gram-negative non-sporing anaerobe
   ii. Principal commensal of large bowel
   iii. Resistant organisms proliferate after broad spectrum antibiotics causing wound infection, intra-abdominal sepsis, and septic shock
   iv. Slow to grow on blood culture and difficult to isolate Laboratory diagnosis may take 10 days
   v. Almost always sensitive to:
      a. Erythromycin
      b. Lincomycin
      c. Chloramphenicol
      d. Clindamycin
      Resistant to penicillin
7. *Clostridium perfringens*

CHEMOTHERAPY

1. Gentamicin (5mg/kg/day) is the antibiotic of first choice. Peak serum concentration (that measured one hour after i.m. injection or 15 min after i.v. injection) should be kept above $5\mu g$/ml
2. In patients not previously hospitalised, *E. coli* is the likely infecting organism and Ampicillin or Cephalosporin may be considered appropriate
3. Chloramphenicol may be useful in uraemic patients
4. Although *pseudomonas aeruginosa* is sensitive to Gentamicin, Carbenicillin may be added if this organism is suspected
5. Gentamicin and Cephalosporin are potentially nephrotoxic
6. *Bacteroides* septicaemia is treated by Lincomycin 600mg i.v. b.d. Intravenous trimethoprim and sulphadimidine has been reported but is not yet critically evaluated

TREATMENT

1. Volume replacement under CVP control, and correction of electrolyte and acid-base balance
2. Antibiotics
3. Surgical treatment of primary infection unless contra-indicated by severe thrombocytopenia and clotting factor deficiency
   i.   Debridement of wounds and burns
   ii. Drainage of abdominal abscess
   iii. Correction of obstruction to biliary, urinary or intestinal tract
   iv. Drainage of septic products of conception or infected post partum uterus. Extensive removal of pelvic organs for salpingitis/parametritis
4. IPPR to correct for as long as possible the pulmonary perfusion defect
5. Management of acute renal failure which may be prerenal, or renal due to glomerular capillary coagulation
6. Heparin, fresh blood, fresh frozen plasma and platelet packs to control DIC and to prevent spontaneous haemorrhage

There is little evidence to support the other therapeutic measures employed

7. Alpha adrenergic blockade
   (Phenoxybenzamine 1 to 2mg/kg at 1mg/min i.v.)
   i. To promote tissue perfusion. Fall in blood pressure corrected by fluid replacement
   ii. In animals, alpha adrenergic blockade abolishes the renal microcoagulopathy occompanying experimental DIC
8. Beta adrenergic stimulation (Isoprenaline 2mg/500ml N. Saline) to improve cardiac function
9. Steroids
   (2 to 6g hydrocortisone per 24 hours by bolus i.v. injection)
   i.   Strong peripheral vaso-dilatory action
   ii. Cell membrane stabilization
   iii. Augmentation of ATP production
   iv. Stabilization of lysosomal membranes
   v.   Prevents absorption of endotoxin into circulation

FURTHER READING

Altemeier, W.A., Todd, J.C. & Inge, W.W. (1967) Gram-negative septicaemia: a growing threat. *Annals of Surgery,* **166,** 530-542.

Daver, B.M. (1971) Septicaemia in the burned patient. *British Journal of Plastic Surgery,* **24,** 280-281.

Lancet (1974) Bacteraemic shock. *Lancet,* i, 296.

MacKenzie, I. & Litton, A. (1974) Bacteroides bacteraemia in surgical patients. *British Journal of Surgery,* **61,** 288-290.

Noone, P., *et al.* (1974) Experience in monitoring Gentamycin therapy during treatment of serious gram-negative sepsis. *British Medical Journal,* i, 477-481.

Abdominal trauma

MECHANISM

Penetrating injury; stab, low velocity missile, high velocity missile

Blunt trauma; especially road traffic accidents

Deceleration

DIAGNOSIS

1. **History**
   - i. Direct trauma of adequate force
   - ii. Of specific loci of pain, e.g. shoulder tip

2. **Examination**
   - i. Tenderness
   - ii. Clinical deterioration, rising pulse, falling BP
   - iii. Increasing girth but may be ileus
   - iv. Patterned abrasions indicate severe trauma
   - v. Associated injuries: ribs, back, pelvis

3. **Investigation**
   - i. Radiographs CXR
     Erect and supine abdomen
   - ii. Contrast radiographs
     - a. Meal for doubtful diaphragmatic rupture
     - b. Studies with water soluble medium for ruptured viscus
     - c. Occasionally arteriography
   - iii. Four quadrant tap may give false negatives
   - iv. Peritoneal lavage
     - a. High degree of accuracy
     - b. Examine for blood and amylase activity

Clinical assessment is readily confused by effects of other injuries, e.g. head or chest, and therefore the abdominal injury may readily be overlooked

MANAGEMENT

Indications for laparotomy:
   - i. Continual shock despite resuscitation
   - ii. Increasing pain and distress
   - iii. Serious suspicion of intra-abdominal injury, e.g. presence of patterned abrasions
   - iv. 'Spleen syndrome' of left shoulder pain, left hypochondrial tenderness with fracture of the left lower ribs
   - v. Free gas or shifting fluid on radiography
   - vi. Blood on four quadrant tap or lavage

MANAGEMENT AT LAPAROTOMY

Laparotomy should be thorough since more than one organ may be involved

1. **Spleen**

   Removal with care not to damage the tail of the pancreas

2. **Bowel**

   Identification may be difficult and may appear just as a small area of pouting mucosa

   Suspicion of injury to the duodenum may necessitate full mobilisation by Kocher's manoeuvre

   Injuries should be resected if necessary and viable bowel anastamosed. In the large bowel a proximal colostomy is frequently advisable

3. **Liver**

   Minor injuries can usually be repaired with simple sutures

   Some major injuries cannot be repaired but if operable hemihepatectomy should be performed at the primary procedure. Bleeding may be controlled temporarily by clamps on the hepatic artery, portal vein and hepatic veins

4. **Vascular**

   Large vessels are rarely injured except by penetrating injury. They may be repaired or grafted primarily if operable.

   Torn mesenteric vessels are often associated with fractures of the lumbar spine. Treatment involves resection of avascular bowel and anastomosis

5. **Pancreas**

   Uncommon injury. Serum amylase is not necessarily raised but amylase may be found with blood in the peritoneal fluid

   Duct tear may be repaired over a small catheter into the duodenum

   Crushed tail may be resected

   Crushed head requires drainage or may even require pancreatico-duodenectomy

   Conservative treatment has a high morbidity rate

FURTHER READING

Attard, J. (1971) Upper retroperitoneal injuries. *British Journal of Surgery,* **58,** 55-60.

Bolton, P.M., Wood, C.B., Quantay, J.B. & Blumgart, L.H. (1973) Blunt abdominal injury. British Journal of Surgery, **60,** 657-663.

Petty, A.H. (1973) Abdominal injuries. *Annals of the Royal College of Surgeons of England,* **53,** 167-177.

Salleh, H.B.M. (1973) Diaphragmatic rupture due to blunt trauma. *British Journal of Surgery,* **60,** 430-433.

Splenectomy

INDICATIONS FOR SPLENECTOMY

1. **Hodgkin's disease and other lymphomas**
   Diagnostic laparotomy in Hodgkin's disease is now the commonest indication for splenectomy
   See Hodgkin's disease, p. 46

2. **Hypersplenism**
   i. Primary hypersplenism. Where abnormal formed elements of the blood are removed inappropriately by a normal spleen
      a. Idiopathic thrombocytopenic purpura
      b. Hereditary spherocytosis
      c. The haemoglobinopathies
   ii. Secondary hypersplenism. Where normal formed elements of the blood are removed inappropriately by an abnormal (usually enlarged) spleen.

3. **Traumatic rupture of spleen**
   An enlarged spleen will rupture more easily than a normal spleen. The enlarged spleens of infective mononucleosis and infective hepatitis have a particularly evil reputation

4. **Where splenectomy is incidental to another surgical procedure**
   i. Radical surgery for gastric carcinoma
   ii. Portal systemic decompression by spleno-renal shunt
   iii. Distal pancreatectomy for chronic pancreatitis or insulinoma

5. **In the treatment of splenic abscess or splenic cyst**
   (Hydatid disease is the commonest cause of splenic cyst)

6. **In giant splenomegaly where symptoms are caused by the size of the spleen**
   i. Myelofibrosis
   ii. Tropical splenomegaly

COMPLICATIONS OF SPLENECTOMY

The incidence and type of complication are closely associated with the indication for splenectomy and the presence of other associated diseases. The high incidence of complication following splenectomy for traumatic rupture is explained by the associated injury to chest and other intra-abdominal organs. Similarly, patients with hypersplenism may be poor operative risks because of anaemia, thrombocytopenia, prolonged steroid therapy or advanced malignant disease.

1. **Haemorrhage**
    i.   From vascular adhesions between the spleen and diaphragm
    ii. Exposure of splenic vessels may be difficult with an enlarged spleen
    iii. In portal hypertension, the retroperitoneal portal-systemic anastomoses make splenectomy particularly difficult
    iv. May occur in the immediate postoperative period from:
         a. Slipped ligature
         b. Oozing. Thrombocytopenia

2. **Subphrenic abscess**
    Routine drainage of splenic bed following all splenectomies is not necessary because the incidence of subphrenic abscess following elective splenectomy alone is less than 1%. Drainage should be considered:
    i.   If haemostasis is not adequate (thrombocytopenia)
    ii. If the tail of pancreas was damaged during splenectomy
    iii. If the trauma caused any pancreatic injury
    iv. If there is a risk of contamination of the splenic bed by gastro-intestinal contents. Such a situation occurs when a spleen is damaged during gastrectomy or colectomy. Similarly, as a result of blunt or penetrating injury, splenic damage can co-exist with an injury to gastro-intestinal tract

3. **Deep vein thrombosis**
    Splenectomy is associated with thrombocythaemia

4. **Portal vein thrombosis**
    If splenectomy was being performed for portal hypertension (hypersplenism or during spleno-renal shunt) then this complication would prevent future portal-caval decompression

5. **Bacterial infection in young children**
    If splenectomy is performed during the first two years of life, there is an increased susceptibility to pyogenic infection, especially pneumococcus or meningococcus

6. **Gastric fistula**
    Can occur if the stomach wall is included in a ligature of the short gastric vessels. Treatment is by drainage of any subphrenic abscess, continuous naso-gastric suction, and parenteral alimentation. Spontaneous closure is awaited

7. **Pancreatic fistula**
    Rarely the tail of the pancreas is damaged during exposure and ligation of splenic vessels

Hodgkin's disease

Survival related to stage and histological grade of tumour

STAGE I

Involvement of single lymph node region
or Involvement of single extra lymphatic organ or site

STAGE II

Two or more lymph node regions involved *on the same side of
        the diaphragm* or
One or more lymph node regions involved and localised
        involvement of extra lymphatic organ *on the same side
        of the diaphragm*

STAGE III

Involvement of lymph node regions on both sides of the
diaphragm

STAGE IV

Disseminated involvement of one or more extra lymphatic sites
with or without associated lymph node involvement

    A No systemic symptoms—more favourable prognosis
    B Systemic symptoms—less favourable prognosis
      Fever
      Sweating
      Weight loss
      Pruritis

HISTOLOGICAL GRADE

    Lymphocytic predominance—favourable prognosis
    Nodular sclerosis—favourable prognosis
    Mixed cellularity—intermediate
    Lymphocytic depletion—ominous prognosis

CYTOLOGY

    Eosinophils
    Lymphocytes
    Histiocytes
    Reed-Sternberg cells
    Areas of fibrosis

SPREAD

By involvement of adjacent lymph nodes or tissues rather than
multicentric origin

INVESTIGATIONS

1. **Adequate surgical biopsy**

2. **Full blood count**
Features of marrow infiltration
  Normochromic, normocytic anaemia
  Leucoerythroblastic anaemia
Features of hypersplenism
  Haemolytic anaemia (with reticulocytosis)
  Leucopenia
  Thrombocytopenia

3. **Liver function tests to include serum alkaline phosphatase**

4. **Chest X-ray**
  Node enlargement, especially superior mediastinum
  Lung parenchyma involvement
  Enlarged cardiac silhouette—pericardial involvement

5. **Skeletal survey or bone scan**
  Deposits preferentially in ribs, spine, pelvis

6. **Lymphangiography**
Abnormal features
  Enlarged nodes
  Abnormal nodal reticular pattern
  Filling defects in nodes
  Abnormal sequence of opacification (shunting around lymphatic obstruction)
  Change in node size and pattern over six months

7. **Myelography (if indicated)**
  To detect extradural deposits

8. **Laparotomy**
  Splenectomy
  Liver biopsy
  Node biopsy
  Assessment of gut involvement
  Oophoropexy

INDICATIONS FOR SPLENECTOMY

1. Accurate staging
   50% patients with Hodgkin's disease have splenic involvement
   25% clinically innocent spleens are involved
2. Protection against marrow depression effects of radiotherapy and chemotherapy
3. Prevention or treatment of hypersplenism
4. Prevention of radiation damage to left kidney and left lung

TREATMENT
Radiotherapy

1. *Supradiaphragmatic Stage I*
'Mantle' irradiation
    Cervical nodes
    Axillary nodes
    Mediastinal nodes
    Normal structures shielded

2. *Supradiaphragmatic Stage II*
'Mantle' irradiation + para-aortic nodes

3. *Infradiaphragmatic nodal disease*
'Inverted–Y' field irradiation
    Para-aortic nodes
    Pelvic nodes
    Inguinal nodes
    ±splenic axis irradiation

4. *Stage IIIA*
Total nodal irradiation. 'Mantle' + 'inverted–Y'

Chemotherapy

Quadruple chemotherapy
    Mustine
    Vinblastine
    Procarbazine
    Prednisone (rapid relief systemic symptoms)
Treatment cycles of six weeks—two weeks of chemotherapy followed by an interlude of four weeks to allow recovery of marrow and gastro-intestinal epithelium. Treatment is continued for three or four cycles after clinical remission. There is no evidence that further maintenance chemotherapy is beneficial

Indications
1. Stage IV
2. Stage IIIB
3. Adjuvant in Stage II or IIIA to provide rapid relief of pressure on vital structures, e.g. Superior vena cava

FURTHER READING
Frei, E. (1974) Combination chemotherapy. *Proceedings of the Royal Society of Medicine,* 67, 425-436.
Irving, M. (1975) The role of surgery in the management of Hodgkin's disease. *British Journal of Surgery,* 62, 853-862.
McElwain, T.J. (1973) The chemotherapy of Hodgkin's disease. *British Journal of Hospital Medicine,* 9, 451-456.
Peckham, M.J. (1973) The radiotherapy of Hodgkin's disease. *British Journal of Hospital Medicine,* 9, 457-468.

Tumour immunology

CANCER RELATED FUNCTION OF RETICULO-ENDOTHELIAL SYSTEM
1. Immunological surveillance
2. 'Antigen processing'
3. Host response to established tumour

1. Immunological surveillance
Mutant cells capable of producing cancer are recognised as 'non-self' and destroyed. Evidence:
  i. Peak incidence of cancer (early life and old age) occurs when immune system is least effective.
  ii. Immuno-suppressive therapy accompanied by an increased risk of cancer (Lymphoma in renal transplant patients)
  iii. Immune deficient diseases accompanied by an increased risk of cancer.

2. 'Antigen processing'
Thymus derived lymphocytes (T cells) important in immunological surveillance, recognise foreign antigens resulting in lymphocyte cytotoxicity and elimination of the antigen

3. Host response to established tumour
  i. *Humoral immune mechanism.* Specific antibodies have been demonstrated in tumours including melanoma, osteosarcoma and neuroblastoma. In melanoma it has been shown that dissemination of tumour beyond regional lymph nodes is anteceded by the disappearance of antibodies from the serum.
  ii. *Cell mediated immune mechanism.* A better differentiation of tumour and an improved prognosis is associated with lymphocyte infiltration (e.g. lip, colon, breast, neuroblastoma). In neuroblastoma an improved prognosis is associated with systemic lymphocytosis.

IMMUNODIAGNOSIS

An increasing number of solid tumours are known to produce macro-molecules which are claimed to be tumour specific antigen (TSA) or tumour associated antigen (TAA). If this is proven then a mechanism will exist not only for early diagnosis and detection of recurrence but also for specific immunother-apy.

1.   Carcinoembryonic antigen (CEA)

Found in the plasma in many malignant tumours including breast, bronchus, gastro-intestinal tract, urothelium

Colo-rectal carcinoma
  i.   CEA is raised in malignant, inflammatory, and infective diseases of the large bowel
       Therefore unlikely to be useful for mass screening
  ii. A serum concentration over 100 ng/ml in a diagnosed carcinoma suggests metastatic disease and a poor prognosis
  iii. Serial estimations will detect tumour recurrence and antecede the clinical appearance of metastases by up to 29 months
  iv. Should a rising CEA titre following potentially curative surgery be regarded as an indication for chemotherapy?

Urothelial carcinoma
  i.   Serum estimations may be useful in screening industrial 'high risk' groups
  ii. Serial serum estimations will recognise tumour recurrence earlier than clinical methods
  iii. Urinary CEA is of little value. It is raised in only 70% of patients with bladder cancer and is raised in infections of the urinary tract

2.   Human chorionic gonadotrophin (radioimmunoassay)
  i.   Detects choriocarcinoma in patients with hydatidiform mole
  ii. Detects early recurrences
  iii. Monitors response to chemotherapy

3.   Alpha fetoprotein (AFP)
  i.   Rate of detection of AFP in primary hepatocullular carcinoma by radioimmunoassay approaches 90%
  ii. Lower levels of AFP can be found in infective hepatitis, cirrhosis, and metastatic hepatic carcinoma
  iii. Carcinoma of stomach, ovary and testis (without hepatic metastases) can produce AFP

IMMUNOTHERAPY

The host response to cancer depends on a complex ill-understood interplay between cell-mediated and humoral immune mechanisms

1. **The enhancement of non-specific immune mechanisms**
    i. Bacterial infection. Noted that when cancer surgery was complicated by infection, the prognosis was improved
    ii. BCG
        a. Maintains remission in acute lymphoblastic leukaemia which has been achieved by chemotherapy
        b. Metastatic nodules of malignant melanoma decrease in size when injected with BCG

2. **Specific active immunotherapy**
    i. Immunisation of patients in remission from acute lymphoblastic leukaemia by allogenic, irradiated, pooled lymphoblasts is effective in maintaining remission
    ii. Immunisation of patients with acute myelogenous leukaemia by intradermal irradiated tumour cells and BCG lengthens remission significantly
    iii. Immunisation of patients with their own irradiated melanoma cells has been shown to produce tumour-specific cytotoxic antibodies, but with no effect of the course on the disease

3. **Specific passive immunotherapy**
    Passive transfer of specifically sensitized pig lymph node cells to patients with advanced malignant disease produces tumour necrosis

FURTHER READING

Currie, G.A. (1972) Human cancer and immunology. *British Journal of Hospital Medicine,* **8**, 685-692.

Feneley, R.C.L. *et al.* (1974) The treatment of advanced breast cancer with sensitized pig lymphocytes. *British Journal of Surgery,* **61**, 825-827.

Hamilton Fairley, G (1971) Immunity to malignant disease in man. *British Journal of Hospital Medicine,* **6**, 633-644.

Lewis, M.G., McCloy, E. & Blake, J. (1973) The significance of humoral antibodies in the localization of human malignant melanoma. *British Journal of Surgery,* **60**, 443-446.

Mathé, G. *et al.* (1969) Active immunotherapy for acute lymphoblastic leukaemia. *Lancet,* i, 697-699.

Symes, M.O. (1974) Tumour immunology. *British Journal of Surgery,* **61**, 929-938.

Symes, M.O. & Riddell, A.G. (1973) The use of immunised pig lymph-node cells in the treatment of patients with advanced malignant disease. *British Journal of Surgery,* **60**, 176-180.

'Early' breast cancer

When there is no clinical, biochemical, radiological and scintigraphic evidence of dissemination beyond T2N1 (see below)

T.N.M. CLASSIFICATION

T—Primary tumour

T 0	No demonstrable tumour
T 1 S	Carcinoma *in situ*
	Non-infiltrating intraduct carcinoma
	Paget's disease of nipple without tumour
T 1	Tumour diameter 2 cm or less without fixation
T 2	Tumour diameter 2 to 5 cm without fixation
T 3	Tumour diameter greater than 5 cm
T 4	Direct extension of a tumour of any size to skin or chest wall (Including peau d'orange)

(Skin tethering and nipple retraction does not affect T classification)

N—Regional lymph nodes

N 0	No palpable homolateral axillary nodes
N 1	Mobile homolateral axillary nodes
N 2	Fixed homolateral axillary nodes
N 3	Homolateral supraclavicular, infraclavicular nodes or oedema of arm

M—Distant metastases

M 0	No distant metastases
M 1	Distant metastases

SCREENING FOR BREAST CANCER

1. Physical examination detects 2 cases every 1000 women examined
2. Physical examination and mammography detect 13.2 cases every 1000 women examined
3. Cancers detected by screening are associated with a lower incidence of lymph node metastases and improved survival rate following treatment

4. Xeroradiography is the most accurate of all screening procedures because of the improved diagnostic quality of the radiographs.
   The radiation dose is significantly lower than mammography.
   Carcinomas demonstrate calcification, an irregular outline with radiating tentacles

5. Screening is of special relevance to patients predisposed to breast cancer
   i.   A family history of breast cancer
   ii.   Carcinoma of the contralateral breast
   iii. Gross fibrocystic disease
   iv.   Past history of intraduct papilloma
   v.   Childless women and those conceiving after 30 years of age
   vi.   A past history of endometrial cancer

Venet, L., Strax, P., Venet, W. & Shapiro, S. (1971) Mass screening for breast cancer. *Cancer,* **28,** 1546-1551.

DETECTION OF OCCULT DISTANT METASTASES

1. Scintigraphy
Between 50 and 70% of bone must be invaded before a metastasis shows up on conventional X-ray. Isotopes (^{18}F, ^{99}Tc—diphosphonate) are taken up preferentially by the osteoid reaction stimulated by metastatic bone deposits
Skeletal metastases can be detected by bone scan in 25% of women who would otherwise be thought to have early breast cancer

Galasko, C.S.B. (1969) The detection of skeletal metastases from mammary cancer by gamma camera scintigraphy. *British Journal of Surgery,* **56,** 757-764.

2. Urinary hydroxyproline estimation
Urinary hydroxyproline is derived from metastatic degradation of newly synthesised collagen. Elevation of hydroxyproline may antecede radiological demonstration of bone metastases by several months. Elevated hydroxyproline also occurs in acromegaly, hyperthyroidism, hyperparathyroidism

Cuschieri, A. (1973) Urinary hydroxyproline excretion in early and advanced breast cancer. *British Journal of Surgery,* **60,** 800-803.

3. Plasma calcitonin
Breast carcinomas can produce calcitonin. Plasma calcitonin may be useful in staging breast carcinoma

Coombes, R.C. *et al.* (1975) Secretion of immunoreactive calcitonin by human breast carcinomas. *British Medical Journal,* iv, 197-199.

RADICAL MASTECTOMY

Conservative radical mastectomy (Patey)
Standard radical mastectomy (Halsted)

1. The main argument for radical mastectomy is that local recurrence is low at 10 to 15%
2. The cosmetic and functional result is better with CRM than SRM. Recurrence within pectoralis major is extremely rare
3. Access to the apex of axilla is easier with SRM than CRM
4. The incidence of involvement of internal mammary nodes in 'early' (defined above) breast cancer
    i. Internal mammary nodes are invaded in 20% of cases
    ii. Medial and central breast tumours involve the internal mammary nodes twice as often as lateral tumours
    iii. Of those patients with invaded axillary nodes, 50% will also have internal mammary node invasion
    iv. Internal mammary node invasion is improbable in T1N0 carcinomata when the primary is in the outer half of the breast and where axillary nodes are subsequently proven to be histologically free of metastases

Handley, R.S. (1975) Carcinoma of the breast. *Annals of the Royal College of Surgeons of England,* **57,** 59-66.

Radical and supraradical procedures do not improve survival rate. Evidence exists that less radical surgery with or without radiotherapy gives comparable survival

SIMPLE MASTECTOMY

In a trial comparing simple mastectomy and radiotherapy with extended radical mastectomy (excision of internal mammary nodes) without radiotherapy, no difference in survival, local or distal recurrence was detected up to 10 years after surgery

Kaae, S. & Johansen, H. (1969) Simple mastectomy plus post operative irradiation by the method of McWhirter for mammary carcinoma. *Annals of Surgery,* **170,** 895-899.

LESSER PROCEDURES

1. **Sector mastectomy and radiotherapy**
    i. Survival at 5 years and 10 years comparable with other methods of treatment
    ii. Local recurrence rate 18%. Of these, a disproportionately high number had axillary node involvement at presentation and a tumour of poor histological grade

(Sector mastectomy, tumour assessment, and radiotherapy may prevent unnecessary mastectomies. Unfavourable histological criteria at tumour assessment would indicate further local surgery)

Taylor, H., Baker, R., Forth, R.W. & Hermon-Taylor, J. (1971) Sector mastectomy in selected cases of breast cancer. *British Journal of Surgery,* **58,** 161-163.

2.'Tylectomy' (wide local excision) and radiotherapy V. Radical mastectomy and radiotherapy

i.   In those patients with clinically involved axillary nodes, the survival was shorter, local and distal recurrence greater in those patients having wide local excision

ii. In those patients without clinically involved axillary nodes, the survival and distal recurrence was comparable but local recurrence was significantly higher with wide local excision

Atkins, H., Hayward, J.L., Klugmann, D.J. & Wayte, A.B. (1972) Treatment of early breast cancer: a report after ten years of clinical trial. *British Medical Journal,* ii, 423-429.

If several suggested techniques give the same expectation of life, it is then necessary to define which of them gives the best chance of local control of the disease so that even though the patient may die of disseminated cancer she is at least saved the pain and suffering of local ulceration.

British Medical Journal (1972) Treatment of early carcinoma of breast. *British Medical Journal,* ii, 417-418.

THE PLACE OF POSTOPERATIVE RADIOTHERAPY

The evidence strongly suggests that postoperative radiotherapy following simple or radical mastectomy has no effect on survival. It may even be harmful to women under 45 years with no axillary metastases

Anderson, J.M. (1973) A critique of the first treatment of carcinoma of the breast. *Surgery, Gynecology and Obstetrics,* **136,** 801-808.

In the largest controlled clinical study so far undertaken on the management of early cancer of breast in women, simple mastectomy and radiotherapy was compared with simple mastectomy alone. There was no difference in survival or the incidence of distant metastases. However, radiotherapy did reduce the incidence of local recurrence.

An international multicentre trial (1976) Management of early cancer of the breast. *British Medical Journal,*i, 1035-1038.

THE PLACE OF ADJUVANT CHEMOTHERAPY

A regimen of cyclophosphamide, methotrexate and 5-fluorouracil has been shown to lengthen the disease-free interval following surgery in early breast cancer. Detection of improved survival must await longer follow up. Slender benefits would have to be weighed against complications of such aggressive chemotherapy—alopecia, cystitis etc.

Bonadonna, G. *et al.,* (1976) Combination chemotherapy as an adjuvant treatment in operable breast cancer. *New England Journal of Medicine,* **294,** 405-410.

Advanced breast cancer

INCLUDES
1. Any breast cancer staged beyond T2N1 at presentation (see p. 52)
2. Recurrent local disease
3. Metastatic disease

PATIENTS LIKELY TO RESPOND TO HORMONE MANIPULATION
1. Those with a long metastasis-free interval
2. Those who have shown a good response to previous hormone therapy
3. Those over 5 years past menopause at presentation of primary
4. Those with advanced local disease without metastasis
5. Those with primarily osseous metastases rather than soft tissue metastases
6. Those with oestrogen receptor-positive tumours

Engelsman, E., Persijn, J.P., Korsten, C.B. & Cleton, F.J. (1973) Oestrogen receptor in human breast cancer tissue and response to endocrine therapy. *British Medical Journal*, ii, 750-752.

TREATMENT OF ADVANCED BREAST CANCER
1. Simpler hormonal manipulation
2. Major endocrine ablation
3. Radiotherapy
4. Chemotherapy
5. Surgical relief of specific complications

1. Simpler hormonal manipulation
(Earliest sign of remission may take two months)

i. Oophorectomy
Premenopausal patients
Early post menopausal patients
Tumour remission rate approximately 30%

ii. Oestrogen therapy
Post menopausal women without evidence of oestrogen secretion
Tumour remission rate increases with increasing years past menopause (30-40%)
Oestrogen continued until tumour reactivation
Second remission on stopping oestrogen in 30% of responders

iii.   Androgen therapy
   Secondary hormonal therapy
   Failed remission or tumour reactivation following
   oophorectomy or oestrogen therapy
iv.   Corticosteroid therapy
   Effect independent of age and menopausal status
   Treatment of hypercalcaemia
   Benefits pain from osseous metastases
   Decreases oedema around cerebral and pulmonary
   metastases
   Induces feeling of well-being
v.   Nafoxidine
   Synthetic, non-steroid antioestrogen

Bloom, H.J.G. & Boesen, E. (1974) Antioestrogens in treatment of breast cancer: value of nafoxidine in 52 advanced cases. *British Medical Journal,* ii, 7-10.

2.   Major endocrine ablation
   Only 30% of patients show objective response
   No improved survival from early major ablation
   Average remission in patients who respond is 18 months
   Contra-indicated in absence of objective response to simpler
   hormonal manipulation
Methods of major endocrine ablation:
i.   Bilateral adrenalectomy
   Major surgical procedure
   Fluid and electrolyte (Na+) problems post-operatively
   Permanent deficient response to 'stress'
ii.   Hypophysectomy
   Hypophysectomy easier to manage than adrenalectomy
   Renin—angiotensin—aldosterone mechanism intact
   Better response to 'stress' (adrenal medulla intact)
   Diabetes insipidus controlled by pitressin until pituitary stalk
   secretes ADH
   a.   Transcranial hypophysectomy:
      Major neurosurgical procedure
      Significant morbidity and mortality
      Unsuitable as a routine procedure
   b.   Trans-sphenoidal hypophysectomy:
      Safer operation
      Small risk of morbidity and mortality:
         Meningitis
         Persistent C.S.F. rhinorrhoea.

c. Isotope implantation ^{90}Y
Transnasal trans-sphenoidal approach
Transethmo-sphenoidal approach
Minor procedure
Ablation often imcomplete. Reimplantation feasible
Radiation damage to:
Diaphragma sellae—CSF rhinorrhoea,
meningitis
Optic chiasma—visual field defects
Oculomotor nerve—oculomotor paralysis

3. Radiotherapy

i. To control locally advanced breast cancer without metastases
ii. To control pain of localised bone metastases
iii. To control localised skin and node metastases
iv. To control signs of mediastinal and spinal cord compression
v. Following internal fixation of pathological fracture

4. Chemotherapy

Cyclical combination chemotherapy

Canellos, G.P. *et al.* (1974) Cyclical combination chemotherapy for advanced breast carcinoma. *British Medical Journal,* i, 218-220.

Canellos, G.P. *et al.* (1976) Combination chemotherapy for advanced breast cancer: response and effect on survival. *Annals of Internal Medicine,* **84**. 389-392.

Intracavitary alkylating agents

5. Surgical relief of specific complications

i. Laminectomy for spinal cord compression
ii. Prophylactic internal fixation of bone metastases

Fidler, M. (1973) Prophylactic internal fixation of secondary neoplastic deposits in long bones. *British Medical Journal,* i, 341-343.

iii. Treatment of pathological fracture by internal fixation

ACUTE PROGRESSIVE HYPERCALCAEMIA IN ADVANCED BREAST CANCER

Recent severe increase in skeletal pain
Recent deterioration in general condition
Symptoms of hypercalcaemia:
Anorexia, nausea, vomiting
Progressive weakness
Lethargy → coma

Treatment
   I.V. saline—corrects dehydration
                calcium diuresis
   Inorganic phosphate therapy. Oral or i.v.
Thalassinus, N. & Joplin, G.F. (1968) Phosphate treatment of hypercalcaemia
due to carcinoma. *British Medical Journal,* iv, 14-19.
   Corticosteroids
   (Calcitonin)
   Discontinue any recently commenced hormonal therapy
   Pituitary ablation
Ominous prognosis

Abdominal aortic aneurysm

INDICATIONS FOR SURGERY

1. Pain. This indicates imminent rupture
2. Recurring peripheral embolisation
3. As a salvage procedure following rupture. These will be cases of extra peritoneal rupture when the expanding haematoma is contained by the posterior peritoneum. Intraperitoneal rupture is usually immediately fatal.
4. Opinion differs on the indication for surgery to asymptomatic aneurysms. The natural history of an aneurysm is to dilate and rupture. Therefore elective surgery should be offered to patients under 70 years with large aneurysms who are otherwise fit for major arterial reconstruction.

SURGICAL PRINCIPLES

1. Involvement of the aorta at the level of the renal arteries may dictate against surgery.
2. The aneurysmal sac may be adherent to inferior vena cava (IVC), iliac veins, duodenojejunal flexure (DJF), or left renal vein (LRV). These may be damaged during the dissection to give proximal and distal control. The LRV can be sacrificed but adherence of DJF may make the aneurysm inoperable.
3. The graft is preclotted before systemic or local heparin is given.
4. Excision of the aneurysmal sac is dangerous because damage to adherent veins will cause profuse haemorrhage. The graft may be laid inside the aneurysm and the anterior wall closed over the graft to prevent bowel adhesion. Otherwise, if the aneurysm has eroded the vertebral bodies, the sac can be sutured behind the graft to provide a bed.
5. Most abdominal aortic aneurysms can be replaced by a tubed Dacron graft. Depending on the distal extent of a compound aneurysm (one involving the aorta and iliac arteries) an aorto-iliac or aorto-femoral bifurcation graft will be necessary for reconstruction. In the case of aorto-femoral bypass, the femoral anastomosis should be end-to-side to allow retrograde flow along the external iliac artery. The pelvic colon will then continue to receive its arterial supply from the internal iliac artery.

6. Dacron grafts should be sutured under light tension to prevent kinking. The shorter the stem of the bifurcation graft the more acute will be the angle between the bifurcating limbs. Kinking at the bifurcation is then prevented.
7. Backflow from the distal arteries should be checked before final suture of the graft. Thrombectomy may be necessary.
8. Staged release of the proximal clamp is practised to prevent hypotension. (Hypotension being related to bleeding from the graft, anoxic vasodilation in the legs, and metabolic acidosis as products of anaerobic respiration are released into the circulation).

FURTHER READING
Wyatt, A.P. (1976) Presentation and management of aneurysms. *Annals of the Royal College of Surgeons of England,* **58**, 52-61.

Methods of arterial reconstruction

HOMOGRAFTS

1. Functioned as a non-viable arterial conduit
2. Aortic replacement was compatible with good long-term results
3. Poor results with peripheral homografts because of thrombosis, arterial degeneration or aneurysm formation

ENDARTERECTOMY

1. Removal of media and atheromatous core leaving external elastic lamina as flow surface
2. Recurrent stenosis in femoral popliteal segment in as many as 50% cases within 2 years (as compared with less than 5% in aorto-iliac segment.) Attempts to provide a smoother flow surface by pressurised gas or fluid endarterectomy have not improved the results.
3. Ideal for localised block in aorto-iliac segment, the arteriotomy being closed with or without a Dacron patch
4. Intimal dissection prevented at distal extremity of endarterectomy by fine axial sutures

AUTOGENOUS VEIN GRAFT

1. Is the arterial replacement of choice below the inguinal ligament, especially over joint lines, for traumatic, aneurysmal or obliterative disease
2. Some series of femoral-popliteal by-pass by reversed autogenous vein show a 70% graft patency at 3 years. About 25% of patients will have a vein of inadequate calibre (4 mm or less) when a composite procedure can be performed using vein to cross the knee joint with endarterectomy or synthetic graft proximally
3. The popliteal 'run-off' is critical to the success of vein by-pass and is considered good when two branches of the popliteal trifurcation are patent
4. Changes in reversed autogenous saphenous vein used for femoral popliteal by-pass
   i. Generalised graft narrowing is the commonest abnormality:
      a. true subendothelial hypertrophy
      b. intimal clot deposition and organisation
   ii. Atherosclerosis involves the vein by-pass in less than 10% of cases

   iii.   'Traumatic stenosis' in para-anastomotic region
         related to the application of holding clamps during
         suturing of the anastomosis
   iv.   Fibrotic changes at the site of the defunctioned
         valves causing narrowing
   v.   Narrowing of the graft by sutures placed too close to
         the parent vein during ligation of tributaries
5. Saphenous vein by-pass *in situ*
   i.   Blood velocity increases as the conducting vessel
         narrows. Therefore velocity is maximal through the
         distal more critical anastomosis, tending to maintain
         patency
   ii.   The vasa vasorum are intact and the nutrition of the
         in-situ graft is normal
   iii. By-pass can be performed to below the popliteal
         trifurcation because the vessels for anastomosis will
         be similar in diameter
   iv.   Kinking and twisting of the graft cannot happen
   v.   Perforating tributaries of the vein must be ligated to
         prevent A-V fistulae
   vi.   Valves are destroyed by passing a vein stripper
         retrogradely or by excision through transverse
         venotomies

SYNTHETIC ARTERIAL GRAFTS
Woven and knitted Dacron
See Implants of non-biological materials, Textiles,p.102
Complications
   1. Haemorrhage
        Minimised by pre-clotting the graft before heparinisation
   2. Suture-line aneurysm
        Occurs as a late complication when silk sutures are used,
        but rarely occurs with non-absorbable synthetic arterial
        sutures
   3. Infection
      i.   Prophylactic antibiotics may have a place in
            preventing this disasterous complication
      ii.   May present with fever, secondary haemorrhage, or
            distal septic emboli
      iii. Invariably the graft must be removed and a
            replacement implanted in a non-infected bed
         a.   An aorto-iliac bifircation graft can be replaced by an
              unilateral axillary bilateral common femoral by-pass
         b.   A femoral popliteal graft can be replaced by a graft
              from external iliac artery to distal popliteal artery via
              the obturator foramen

4. *Graft failure*
    i.   Synthetic grafts are less favourable than reversed autogenous vein where:
         a.   Blood flow is reduced
         b.   There is angulation across joint lines
         c.   The graft is anastomosed to small arteries

THE HEALING OF SYNTHETIC ARTERIAL GRAFTS

1. Endothelialisation from the host artery to a maximum of 10 mm
2. Fibroblasts and vascular granulation tufts invade the wall of the graft organising the thrombus. Unfortunately the thrombus of the flow surface is not totally invaded so that endothelialisation is incomplete
3. Especially over a joint line, the distortion of synthetic fibre bundles with movement crushes the healing tissues as they invade the interstices. There is discontinuity of the flow surface pseudo-intima at that point predisposing to pseudo-intimal dissection, thrombosis, or degenerative changes
4. Attempts to encourage greater healing of grafts have involved design of grafts with greater porosity
5. Further advance towards full wall healing and endothelialisation of the flow surface has been claimed by replacing the tightly-knitted smooth fibre bundles of conventional grafts with loosely-knitted bundles of highly texturised yarn combined with an integral external velour component (Filamentous velour knitted Dacron)

FURTHER READING
Helsby, R. & Moosa, A.R. (1975) Aorto-iliac reconstruction with special reference to the extraperitoneal approach. *British Journal of Surgery,* **62**, 596-600.
Taylor, G.W. (1973) Chronic arterial occlusion. In *Peripheral Vascular Surgery,* ed. Birnstingl, M. pp211-234, William Heinemann.
Watt, J.K., Gillespie, G., Pollock, J.G. & Reid, W. (1974) Arterial surgery in intermittent claudication. *British Medical Journal,* i, 23-26.

Profundoplasty

THE PROFUNDA FEMORIS ARTERY (PFA)

1. The PFA is the artery of supply to the thigh and its terminal branches anastomose with the muscular branches of the popliteal artery and with the cruciate anastomosis. A collateral network therefore exists for bypass of an occluded superficial femoral artery.
2. When the PFA is involved in atheromatous degeneration the plaque is usually constant in position on the posterior wall of the artery. The plaque will not be demonstrated by arteriography unless lateral or oblique views of the PFA are obtained.
3. The artery is rarely occluded by atheroma.
4. The medial and lateral circumflex arteries usually arise within centimetres of the origin of PFA and their branches contribute to the trochanteric and cruciate anastomosis. Therefore even when the origin of the PFA is occluded the artery below the circumflex branches is kept patent by these anastomoses.

INDICATIONS FOR PROFUNDOPLASTY

1. In those patients with rest pain and ischaemic ulceration where femoral-popliteal bypass is not possible because of a poor 'run-off' at the trifurcation of the popliteal artery, and where narrowing or occlusion of the PFA has been demonstrated by arteriography.
2. In those patients with rest pain and ischaemic ulceration where the arterial tree is suitable for femoral-popliteal bypass but where the general condition of the patient dictates against a lengthy and major procedure. Profundoplasty is swifter and can often be performed under local anaesthetic.
3. In those patients with established gangrene making amputation at some level inevitable but where it is considered that an improvement in calf or ankle blood flow will either allow a more conservative amputation or improve the healing potential of a below-knee amputation.
4. In those patients with significant aorto-iliac disease and an occluded superficial femoral artery, profundoplasty should be performed at the same time as aorto-iliac endarterectomy or bypass

METHODS OF PROFUNDOPLASTY

1. Endarterectomy

i.   When atheroma involves only the orifice, the PFA can be 'unplugged' from an arteriotomy in the common femoral artery

ii. When a longer length of PFA is involved the artery should be dissected distally (for up to 20 cm) until soft, pliable arterial wall is reached. The atheroma is then removed by open or closed endarterectomy:

    a.   Open endarterectomy in continuity with the common femoral artery with vein patch closure of the longitudinal arteriotomy

    b.   Closed endarterectomy from an arteriotomy in the common femoral artery. This can be supplemented (if necessary) by a low profunda arteriotomy closed by vein patch. This method is particularly useful when the procedure is performed at the same time as aorto-ilial bypass—the common femoral arteriotomy being used for anastomosis of the Dacron bifurcation graft.

2. Bypass

From the aorta or iliac arteries to the PFA beyond the block by synthetic graft or reversed autogenous vein

One of the most accurate methods of evaluating improvement in peripheral blood flow is to measure ankle blood pressure (by Doppler method) and to monitor its relationship to exercise. An increased peripheral blood flow is characterised by:

1.   An increase in resting ankle pressure
2.   An increase in claudicating distance
3.   A smaller fall in ankle pressure in response to exercise
4.   A more rapid return to resting ankle pressure

Objective improvement following profundoplasty can only be demonstrated when the procedure is performed for severe claudication, rest pain or ischaemic ulceration. Intermittent claudication is rarely abolished and the procedure should not be considered as an alternative to femoral-popliteal bypass.

FURTHER READING

Kiely, P.E., Lumley, J.S.P. & Taylor, G.W. (1973) Extended endarterectomy of the profunda femoris artery *Archives of Surgery*, **106**, 605-609.

Martin, P., Renwick, S. & Stephenson, C. (1968) On the surgery of the profunda femoris artery. *British Journal of Surgery*, **55**, 539-542.

Arterial injury

AETIOLOGY
1. Penetrating injury
   i. Knife, gunshot
   ii. High velocity missile
2. Blunt trauma or crushing injury
3. Fracture or dislocation
   i. Supracondylar fracture of the humerus and the brachial artery
   ii. Fracture of neck of humerus and the axillary artery
   iii. Posterior dislocation of the knee and the popliteal artery
   iv. Clavicular fracture and the subclavian artery etc.
4. Acute deceleration injury
   Aortic tear at the junction of arch and descending aorta
5. Traction injury
   Acute lateral flexion of cervical spine associated with motorcycle accidents may produce brachial plexus and subclavian artery injury
6. Following arterial cannulation

ARTERIAL DAMAGE
1. Incomplete or complete laceration of arterial wall
2. Intimal tear, intimal flap, intimal dissection with local and propagated thrombosis
3. Contusion of the arterial wall
4. Incomplete laceration of arterial wall and false aneurysm formation
5. Injury to adjacent artery and vein with arterio-venous fistula formation
6. Actual tissue loss from high velocity missiles

PRINCIPLES OF MANAGEMENT
1. Signs of arterial occlusion is an indication for immediate exploration. Delay is associated with an increased amputation rate
2. In the absence of obvious signs, diagnosis depends on suspicion. The most subtle signs of distal ischaemia must be sought for in the context of the nature of injury, site of fracture etc. A pulse distally does not exclude the possibility of arterial injury

3. Arteriography is not necessary when signs of distal ischaemia are present but should be performed early if suspicion exists
4. Penetrating injury in the region of major vessels should be explored even in the absence of ischaemia, to prevent false aneurysm and arterio-venous fistula formation
5. Arterial spasm should *not* be diagnosed unless structural arterial damage has been excluded by surgical exploration. Sudden narrowing and loss of pulsation of an artery is probably caused by intimal damage and thrombosis at that point rather than arterial spasm. An arteriotomy should be performed at the point of narrowing.

SURGICAL PRINCIPLES

1. Proximal control of the artery with or without systemic or local heparinisation
2. Proximal and distal catheter thrombectomy
3. Arterial reconstruction
   i. Direct suture of an incomplete laceration or end-to-end anastomosis of a complete arterial laceration. Proximal and distal mobilisation of the artery may be necessary for end-to-end anastomosis without tension, but collateral branches should never be sacrificed
   ii. Excision of a length of contused or severely lacerated artery. Restoration of continuity by reversed autogenous vein graft
   iii. Intimal fracture or flap is treated by arteriotomy, tacking down of the intima with fine, axial mattress sutures and vein patch angioplasty
   iv. If an arterio-venous fistula has formed, the artery and vein are repaired and a muscle or fascial flap interposed to prevent recurrence. A distal arterio-venous fistula can be treated by quadruple ligation
4. Venous thrombectomy and venous reconstruction should be performed if a major vein is damaged and thrombosed
5. Fasciotomy is often advocated as routinely necessary following arterial repair. Venous compression caused by increase in tissue pressure will be prevented
6. Internal fixation of an unstable fracture should be performed at the same time as arterial reconstruction. Not essential if a reduced fracture is stable (supracondylar fracture of humerus, transverse fracture of tibia etc.)
7. Prosthetic graft as arterial replacement in penetrating arterial injury is contra-indicated because of the danger of sepsis and secondary haemorrhage.

FALSE ANEURYSM OF SUPERIOR MEDIASTINUM

Acute deceleration injury can tear the aorta at the junction of arch with descending aorta where the latter is fixed by intercostal arteries. In a proportion of these patients the haematoma will be contained by the integrity of the overlying pleura. Diagnosis depends upon suspicion, recognition of delayed or weak femoral pulses, a widened superior mediastinum and, definitively, aortography.

Treatment is by left-atrium to femoral by-pass and resection with grafting. Rarely the haematoma around a partial tear of the aorta will organise to a traumatic aneurysm.

FURTHER READING
Slaney, G. & Ashton, F. (1971) Arterial injuries and their management. *Postgraduate Medical Journal,* **47**, 257-269.

Methods of investigation of the thyroid

1. MECHANICAL EFFECTS

 i. Clinically—degree of stridor
 ii. Radiographically—air or contrast laryngography and tracheography
 iii. Endoscopically

2. SITES OF ACTIVITY

Scanning or gamma camera pictures of areas of radioactive iodine uptake

3. FUNCTION

Indirect

 i. *Basal metabolic rate.* Measurement of energy output under resting conditions by measuring the oxygen uptake and standardising the result with reference to surface area. An investigation which is difficult technically and prone to many inaccuracies
 ii. *Blood cholesterol.* A presumptive diagnosis of hypothyroidism is made if the level is over 8mmol/l (300mg/100ml) if other causes of hypercholesterolaemia may be excluded

Direct

 i. *Protein bound iodine.* Measures bound thyroid hormone levels but is prone to inaccuracy from ingested or administered iodine compounds, especially contrast media, and from variations in the binding globulin levels
 Normal levels 280 to 630nmol/l (3.5 to 8.0 μg/100ml)
 ii. ^{131}I *uptake test.* Tends to be inaccurate because of other interactions. Requires multiple measurements in a specialised laboratory over 2 days
 Normal uptake 20 to 55% in 24 hours
 Plasma clearance 5 to 60ml/min
 iii. ^{132}I *uptake,* ^{99m}Tc *uptake.* Both used because of the lower radiation to the gland
 ^{99m}Tc Normal uptake less than 3% at 20 min

iv. *Thyroid hormones.* Thyroid stimulating hormone, thyroxine and tri-iodothyonine may all be measured in the blood. The number of unoccupied binding sites on thyroxine binding globulin may be estimated by a number of different tests

Estimates of the level of active thyroxine may be obtained by dividing the total thyroxine by the number of unoccupied sites. This figure by various methods is expressed as the effective thyroxine ratio, free thyroxine index or normalised thyroxine ratio

In view of the large overlap of results into the normal range it has been suggested that, in any one patient, initially the level of active thyroxine should be measured which will give some results unequivocally, normal, hyperthyroid or hypothyroid. In borderline hyperthyroid patients the tri-iodothyronine level will help and in borderline hypothyroid patients the thyroid stimulating hormone level will help.

FURTHER READING
Britton, K.E., Quinn, V., Brown, B.L. & Ekins, R.P. (1975) A strategy for thyroid function tests. *British Medical Journal,* iii, 350-352.

Solitary thyroid nodule

Nodules diagnosed clinically as solitary are found to be multiple in 50% cases at surgery or histology

PATHOLOGY
1. Clinically toxic patients usually have a simple adenoma but these form a small group; about 6% of cases
2. The incidence of malignancy is quoted between 6% and 58% (*cf.* nodular goitre 1% to 25%) but in most series at 6% to 12%

INVESTIGATIONS
1. Blood investigations for thyrotoxicosis
2. Soft tissue radiographs of the neck to detect any tracheal compression
3. Isotopic scanning is of little value since both 'cold' and 'warm' nodules have an incidence of malignancy (12.8% and 6% respectively)
4. Lymphography has been found to be of little value
5. Needle biopsy has a risk of tumour implantation in the track
6. Out-patient high-speed drill biopsy can be useful

Sachdeva, H.S., Wig, J.D., Bose, S.M., Chowdhary, G.C. & Dutta, B.N. (1974) The solitary thyroid nodule. *British Journal of Surgery,* **61**, 368-370.

MANAGEMENT
1. Exploration and nodulectomy with wide clearance
2. Hemithyroidectomy. Carefully preserve the recurrent laryngeal nerve and parathyroid with blood supply. This technique ensures clearance of the tumour but with little morbidity. Taking the whole isthmus ensures that no problems arise from compression when the remainder hypertrophies
   Frozen section is only recommended for suspicious lymph nodes
3. Total thyroidectomy for clinically unequivocal carcinoma

FURTHER READING
Messaris, G., Kyriakou, K., Vasilopoulos, P. & Tourtas, C. (1974) The single thyroid nodule and carcinoma. *British Journal of Surgery,* **61**, 943-944.
Psarras, A., Papadopoulos, S.N., Livadas, D., Pharmakiotis, A.D. & Koutras, D.A. (1972) The single thyroid nodule. *British Journal of Surgery,* **59**, 545-548.
Taylor, S. (1969) The solitary thyroid nodule. *Journal of the Royal College of Surgeons of Edinburgh,* **14**, 267-271.

Thyroid cancer

Comprises 0.7% of all malignancies in men and 0.2% in women

AETIOLOGY

i.   Endemic goitre is thought to predispose to thyroid cancer due to the raised TSH level. This has been proved in animals but the statistics in man are mixed
ii. Irradiation, especially at low levels in children, raises the incidence. There may be a 20 year or more latent period
iii. Some forms of medullary carcinoma are familial

PATHOLOGY

i.   Tumours derived from follicular cells may be:
     a. Largely follicular
     b. Largely papillary
     c. Anaplastic
ii. Tumours derived from parafollicular cells are medullary
iii. Lymphomas may present in the thyroid

INCIDENCE

Papillary 48%
Follicular 20%
Anaplastic 25%
Medullary 7%

Johnston, I.D.A. (1975) The surgery of thyroid cancer. *British Journal of Surgery,* **62**, 765-768.

CLINICAL FEATURES

i.   May present with diffuse swelling, nodular swelling or single nodule. Occasionally presents with lymph node involvement or secondary metastases
ii. Presence of cragginess, fixation, hoarseness or Horner's syndrome signify extracapsular spread and worse prognosis
iii. Patients under 30 years tend to have a papillary carcinoma with a good prognosis. Over 50% 10 year survival

Richardson, J.E., Beaugie, J.M., Brown, C.L. & Doniach, I. (1974) Thyroid cancer in young patients in Great Britain. *British Journal of Surgery,* **61**, 85-89.

iv. Follicular carcinoma is rare under 30 years. About 40% 10 year survival

v. Anaplastic carcinoma tends to occur in older patients and has a very poor prognosis with an 8% 10 year survival, most of the deaths being in the first year

vi. Medullary carcinoma is familial in 10% of cases. Early cases in relatives may be detected by a high serum calcitonin. The familial form of medullary carcinoma tends to be associated with phaeochromocytomas and mucosal neuromas

vii. Lymphoma may arise in a pre-existent Hashimoto's thyroiditis. It is very radio-sensitive

DIAGNOSIS

i. The diagnosis is largely on clinical grounds

ii. Scanning is of little value except to detect metastases. 20 to 30% of follicular and papillary carcinomas take up radioactive iodine

iii. Ultrasound may reveal the cystic nature of follicular tumours

iv. Raised calcitonin levels are diagnostic of medullary carcinoma

v. Diagnosis in inoperable cases may be confirmed by needle or high speed drill biopsy. The risk of implantation in the track is, in practice, very small

vi. Thyroid cancer virtually never produces thyrotoxicosis

vii. Differential diagnosis includes: Hashimoto's, de Quervain's and Riedel's thyroiditis

TREATMENT

1. Papillary and follicular tumours

i. Extracapsular thyroidectomy preserving the parathyroids and their blood supply. Frozen section may be necessary for sections of enlarged lymph nodes
If tumour is found then a local lymph node resection is adequate and radical block dissection need not be done—see (ii)

ii. Postoperatively a diagnostic scan is performed and if localised activity is found a therapeutic dose of ^{131}I is given (about 200mCi)

iii. Inoperable cases are treated with ^{131}I if functioning or with external irradiation with high energy electron beams. Secondaries may be treated similarly

2. *Anaplastic tumours*
    i.   Total thyroidectomy as in 1 (i)
    ii. Postoperative irradiation to the neck and upper mediastinum
    iii. Inoperable tumours are irradiated

3. *Medullary tumours*
    i.   Total thyroidectomy
    ii. Irradiation for residual tumour or for inoperable tumour

4. *Lymphomas*
    These are treated like lymphomas elsewhere by biopsy and irradiation including the upper mediastinum in the field

Hormone therapy

Well differentiated tumours in childhood may be TSH dependent and regress if thyroid hormones are administered. Thyroid hormones are given routinely following thyroidectomy. Hormone therapy alone is not employed

Chemotherapy

Chemotherapy may be especially useful in lymphomas. In tumours other than lymphomas it has little part to play at present

Immunotherapy

This is being investigated but has little part to play at present

FURTHER READING

Doniach, I., Dolphin, G.W., Henk, J.M., Taylor, S., Scott, J.S. & Halnan, K.E. (1974) Thyroid cancer. *Proceedings of the Royal Society of Medicine*, **67**, 1103-1108.

Williams, E.D., Wade, J.S.H., Johnston, I.D.A. & Halnan, K.E. (1975) Barber's Company Symposium on malignant disease of the thyroid. *British Journal of Surgery*, **62**, 757-771.

Cryosurgery

CRYOBIOLOGY

The rapid freezing of living cells is cytotoxic because of:
1. Intracellular ice crystal formation
2. Intracellular accumulation of toxic concentrations of electrolytes
3. Denaturation of cell membrane lipid-protein complexes
4. Microvascular stasis and thrombosis

Slow thawing is more damaging then rapid thawing

CRYOSURGERY

1. Closed nitrous oxide (–70°C) cryoprobe is suitable for benign and premaligant lesions. In larger vascular lesions, liquid nitrogen (–180°C) may be necessary to produce cryonecrosis
2. Configuration of cryolesion determined by size and shape of cryoprobe. Depth of cryolesion determined by compression or elevation of cryoprobe against the lesion
3. Adrenaline infiltration decreases vascularity and shortens duration of freezing. Freezing for up to 2 min is sufficient for benign lesions on squamous or mucosal surfaces
4. Biopsy can be taken during thawing
5. A serous discharge (sometimes profuse) follows thawing until a slough or crust forms
6. In benign lesions healing is complete within 2 weeks

ADVANTAGES OF CRYOSURGERY

1. Usually no anaesthetic is required and out-patient treatment is possible
2. Minimal postoperative discomfort because of minimal tissue response and destruction of nerve endings
3. Oedema, infection, primary and secondary haemorrhage is rare
4. Scarring is minimal
5. Often the treatment of choice for benign and premalignant lesions of accessible mucosal surfaces. Useful in palliation of recurrent malignant disease at these sites. (Generally, no place for cryosurgery in the treatment of primary invasive carcinoma)
6. Cryodestruction may initiate a specific immune response

USES OF CRYOSURGERY

1. Benign lesions
i.   Lesions of tongue, floor of mouth, palate and buccal mucosa—papillomas, fibroepithelial polyps, mucous retention cysts, ranulas, fibrous epulides, etc.
ii. Tonsillectomy where haemostasis may be difficult as in blood dyscrasias, haemophilia and von Willebrand's disease
iii. Telangiectases, haemangiomata, and lymphangiomata
  a. Ideal for treating intra-oral lesions when haemorrhage and scarring are avoided
  b. Cryonecrosis of intra-osseous haemangiomata destroys cellular elements of bone, but calcified framework is rapidly repopulated
  c. Cryosurgery useful in arteriovenous malformations of brain and meninges
iv. Warts and condylomata
v.   Second and third degree haemorrhoids
vi. Hypophysectomy either by transcranial or transphenoidal route. (Diabetic retinopathy, advanced breast carcinoma, benign pituitary tumours, etc.)
vii. Cervical erosion
viii. Lens extraction in cataract surgery

2. Premalignant lesions
i.   Leukoplakia. Hyperkeratoses. Bowen's disease
ii. Can be used to remove rectal polyps
iii. Cryonecrosis of walls of bony cavity following currettage of ameloblastomata and dentigerous cysts prevents local recurrence

3. Malignant lesions
i.   Control of recurrent cervical carcinoma in the vault of vagina
ii. In the palliation of residual or recurrent malignancy of the oral cavity. Pain, haemorrhage, tumour size, and secondary infection of necrotic tumour can be controlled
iii. As an alternative to other methods of treating basal cell carcinoma and squamous cell carcinoma of skin
iv. Rarely in the treatment of primary invasive carcinoma of cervix and oral cavity where conventional treatment is contra-indicated by age, debility, etc.

FURTHER READING
Chamberlain, G. (1975) Cryosurgery in gynaecology. *British Journal of Hospital Medicine*, **14**, 26-37.
Farrant, J. (1975) Cryobiology. *British Journal of Hospital Medicine*, **14**, 8-13.
Holden, H.B. & McKelvie, P. (1972) Cryosurgery in the treatment of head and neck neoplasia. *British Journal of Surgery*, **59**, 709-712.
Poswillo, D. (1973) Cryosurgery in and around the oral cavity. In *Recent Advances in Surgery*, No. 8, ed. Selwyn Taylor Ch. 3. Edinburgh and London: Churchill Livingstone.
Poswillo, D. (1975) Cryosurgery in oral surgery. *British Journal of Hospital Medicine*, **14**, 47-54.
Richardson, A. (1975) Cryosurgery in neurosurgery. *British Journal of Hospital Medicine*, **14**, 39-46.
Williams, K.L. & Holden, H.B. (1975) Cryosurgery in general and E.N.T. surgery. *British Journal of Hospital Medicine*, **14**, 14-25.

Deep vein thrombosis; pulmonary embolism

PATHOGENESIS

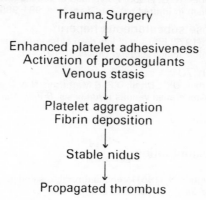

Trauma. Surgery

↓

Enhanced platelet adhesiveness
Activation of procoagulants
Venous stasis

↓

Platelet aggregation
Fibrin deposition

↓

Stable nidus

↓

Propagated thrombus

HIGH RISK GROUPS

1. Previous DVT
2. Previous pulmonary embolus
3. The elderly
4. Malignant disease
5. Extensive trauma. Extensive surgery
6. Obesity
7. Abdominal or pelvic surgery rather than upper limb or head and neck surgery
8. Contraceptive pill
9. Congestive cardiac failure. Myocardial infarction

PROPHYLAXIS

1. Physical means
   i.   Early ambulation
   ii. Electrical stimulation of calf

Browse, N.L. & Negus, D. (1970) Prevention of postoperative leg vein thrombosis by electrical muscle stimulation. An evaluation with 125I-labelled fibrinogen. *British Medical Journal*, iii, 615-618.

   iii. Pneumatic leggings

Hills, N.H. *et al.* (1972) Prevention of deep vein thrombosis by intermittent pneumatic compression of calf. *British Medical Journal*, i, 131-135.

   iv. Foot pedaling machine

Sabri, S., Roberts, V.C. & Cotton, L.T. (1971) Prevention of early postoperative deep vein thrombosis by passive exercise of leg during surgery. *British Medical Journal*, iii, 82-83.

2. Chemical means
    i.   Aspirin—decreases platelet adhesiveness
    ii.   Phenformin—increases fibrinolysis
    iii. Oral anticoagulants

Sevitt, S. & Gallaher, N. G. (1959) Prevention of venous thrombosis and pulmonary embolism in injured patients. *Lancet,* ii, 981-989.

    iv. Low dose subcutaneous heparin

Kakkar, V.V. *et al.* (1972) Efficacy of low dose of heparin in prevention of deep-vein thrombosis after major surgery. *Lancet,* ii, 101-106.

    v.   Dextran 70

Lambie, J.M., Barber, D.C., Dhall, D.P. & Matheson, N.A. (1970) Dextran 70 in prophylaxis of postoperative venous thrombosis. *British Medical Journal,* ii, 144-145.

DIAGNOSIS

1. Clinical examination
Unreliable

Sevitt, S. & Gallagher, N. (1961) Venous thrombosis and pulmonary embolism. *British Journal of Surgery,* **48**, 475-489.

2. Venography
Essential to confirm diagnosis
Essential to delineate extent of thrombus

Thomas, M.L. (1970) Radiological diagnosis of deep vein thrombosis and its sequelae. *Proceedings of the Royal Society of Medicine,* **63**, 123-126.

3. Radioactive fibrinogen (^{125}I)
Preferential uptake by forming thrombus
Greater than 90% correlation with venography
Unreliable above midthigh
Risk of serum hepatitis
Unreliable in presence of haematoma or healing wound

4. Ultrasound flow detector (Doppler effect)
Harmless, can be used in pregnancy
Practical, inexpensive screening method
May give false negative with non-occlusive thrombus
Flow in collateral or superficial vein may mask DVT

Evans, D.S. & Cockett, F.B. (1969) Diagnosis of deep-vein thrombosis with an ultrasonic Doppler technique. *British Medical Journal,* ii, 802-804.

5. Impedance plethysmography

6. Radioactive streptokinase

TREATMENT

1. Anticoagulants
2. Pharmacological fibrinolysis
3. Surgical thrombectomy
4. Vein ligation or plication

Mavor, G.E., Galloway, J.M.D. & Karmody, A.M. (1970) The surgical aspects of deep vein thrombosis. *Proceedings of the Royal Society of Medicine,* **63**, 126-131.

Mavor, G.E. & Galloway, J.M.D. (1969) Iliofemoral venous thrombosis. Pathological considerations and surgical management. *British Journal of Surgery,* **56**, 45-59.

The prevention of pulmonary embolism in surgical patients

1. Dextran 70

Dextran 70 administered pre-operatively prevented, and reduced mortality from, pulmonary embolism
500cc of Dextran 70 given at induction of anaesthesia and 500cc immediately postoperatively

Kleine, A. *et al.* (1975) Dextran 70 in prophylaxis of thromboembolic disease after surgery. *British Medical Journal,* ii, 109-112.

2. Low dose subcutaneous heparin

Calcium heparin (5000u) given pre-operatively and thereafter eight-hourly for seven days. Statistically significant fewer deaths in the heparin group than the control group. No statistical difference in blood loss but an increased incidence of wound haematoma in heparin group.

Lancet (1975) Prevention of fatal postoperative pulmonary embolism by low doses of heparin. An International Multicentre Trial. *Lancet,* ii, 45-51.

Metabolic response to injury

'Trauma'

↓

↑cortisol   ↑catecholamines
↑Aldosterone   ↑growth hormone   ↑glucagon   ↑ADH

↓

Distal tubular reabsorption of sodium
potassium loss

↓

Insulin antagonism
(despite compensatory increased serum insulin)
Extent influenced by:
severity of trauma, operation or burn
presence or absence of sepsis

↓

Intracellular catabolism

↓

Weight loss
Increased urinary nitrogen
Increased urinary potassium

	Normal urinary loss	After moderate uncomplicated trauma
Nitrogen	8 - 10 g/day	10 - 20 g/day
Potassium	70 - 100 mEq/day	100 - 140 mEq/day
Sodium	70 - 100 mEq/day	5 - 20 mEq/day
Water	1500 ml/day	1000 ml/day

Duration approximately one week
(10 g nitrogen ≡ 62 g protein ≡ 300 g muscle tissue)
Negative nitrogen balance is physiological following 'trauma'
but not obligatory, even in severe burns (associated with
massive catabolism) provided sufficient calories are provided

Penalties of prolonged negative nitrogen balance
1. Delayed healing
2. Increased susceptibility to infection
3. Weight loss (if greater than 30% recovery improbable)
4. Hypoproteinaemia
5. Increased mortality

Parenteral feeding

INDICATIONS FOR PARENTERAL FEEDING

1. **Gastro-intestinal failure**
   Prolonged paralytic ileus
   Enteric fistulae
   Chronic intestinal obstruction
   Extensive inflammatory bowel disease
   Acute ulcerative colitis
2. **To supplement oral feeding in:**
   Severe burns
   Massive or prolonged infection
3. **To treat malnutrition pre-operatively**
   Oesophageal carcinoma
   Pyloric stenosis

CALORIE REQUIREMENT

Neonate 100 kcal/kg/day
Adult 40 kcal/kg/day
Adult (severe catabolism) 50-60 kcal/kg/day
Given (approx.) as:
   Carbohydrate 50%
   Fat 30-40%
   Protein 10-15%

CALORIC VALUES

1. Carbohydrate   4 kcal/g
2. Protein   4 kcal/g
3. Fat   9 kcal/g
4. Ethanol   7 kcal/g

1. **Carbohydrate source**
   i. Glucose
   The physiological carbohydrate
   In high concentration may produce hyperosmolar state
   ii. Fructose
   Converted to glucose in liver
   Good liver function therefore essential
   Can produce lactic acidosis in young children and shocked patients
   iii. Sorbitol
   Non physiological
   Converted to fructose in liver
   Potent osmotic diuretic

2. **Protein source**
   i. Casein hydrolysate. Aminsol
   As satisfactory as amino acid preparations and cheaper
   Possibility of allergy to peptides
   ii. Synthetic crystalline amino acid preparations
   Vamin
   Aminoplex
   Trophysan

3. **Fat source**
   Usually emulsions of soya bean oil
   Intralipid 10%— 900 kcal/l
   Intralipid 20%—1800 kcal/l
   Contra-indications
   Liver failure
   Haemorrhagic diathesis
   Especially useful in hypercatabolic states when 40 to 50% of total calorie requirement may be given as Intralipid
   Hyperlipidaemia interferes with blood X-match

COMPLICATIONS

   1. Septicaemia, especially opportunistic gram-positive bacteria and fungi
   2. Thrombophlebitis
   3. Metabolic acidosis
   4. Hyperosmolar state
   5. Deficiencies on prolonged i.v. feeding of:
   Vitamins
   Folic acid
   Minerals: iron, calcium, magnesium, zinc, iodine, manganese, cobalt, copper

COMPOSITE EXAMPLES
1.   Aminosol-Fructose-Ethanol
2.   Vamin 7%
3.   Aminoplex—5

FURTHER READING
Freeman, J.B. & Litton, A.A. (1974) Preponderance of gram-positive infections during parenteral alimentation. *Surgery, Gynecology and Obstetrics,* **139,** 905-908.
Lee, H.A. (1974) Intravenous nutrition. *British Journal of Hospital Medicine,* **11,** 719-728.
Lee, H.A. (1975) Intravenous nutrition. *Annals of the Royal College of Surgeons of England,* **56,** 59-68.
Rodrigues, R.J. & Wolff, W.I. (1974) Fungal septicaemia in surgical patients. *Annals of Surgery,* **180,** 741-747.

Bladder tumours

AETIOLOGY

1. Ingested carcinogens—particularly relevant to the rubber and dye industries since beta-naphthylamine has been shown to cause bladder tumours
2. Animal experiments have suggested that metabolites of tryptophan may induce tumours
3. Smoking may be related

PRESENTATION

1. Haematuria
2. Symptoms of cystitis but with a sterile pyuria
3. Positive cytology on screening in the dye industries

ASSESSMENT

Tumours may arise at multiple primary sites or metastasise throughout the urinary tract therefore the whole tract must be examined

1. Urine culture to diagnose superadded infection and exclude tuberculosis
2. Urine cytology—mainly used for screening
3. Radiography especially intravenous urography which demonstrates:
   i. Tumours in the upper tract
   ii. Filling defect in the bladder if the tumour is over 3 cm diameter
   iii. Involvement of the ureteric orifice
4. Cystoscopy which enables inspection of:
   i. The size and position of the tumour
   ii. The nature of the tumour
   iii. A preliminary assessment of the degree of invasion, necrosis of fronds is an indication of invasion
5. Biopsy for histological grading and detection of muscle invasion
6. Bimanual EUA to assess extent of tumour

PATHOLOGY

1. Benign tumours are very uncommon and to be called such must be composed of entirely normal epithelium
2. Urothelial tumours. Transitional-cell carcinoma is by far the commonest tumour
3. Metaplastic tumours. Squamous cell carcinoma is uncommon
4. Glandular tumours. Adenocarcinoma is rare
5. 'Mossy' bladder epithelium is almost certainly not pre-cancerous

(Miller and Mitchell, 1969)

CLASSIFICATION OF TUMOURS

There are many classification systems: the simplest are based on histological grades and on the TNM system (Nodes are not accessible for assessment except at open operation)

1.   Histology

Grade	Histology	Usual gross appearance
Low	Well differentiated	Fronded
Intermediate	Moderately differentiated	Fronded and solid
High	Poorly differentiated	Solid

2.   TNM system

T_1 Tumour in mucosa and submucosa	Impalpable at EUA
T_2 Invasion of superficial muscle	Rubbery thickening
T_3 Invasion of deep muscle and to serosa	Hard mass, mobile
T_4 Invasion of other viscera or spread to pelvic wall	Hard mass, immobile or fixed

TREATMENT OF TRANSITIONAL-CELL CARCINOMA

1. **Superficial lesions $T_{1, 2}$ and some T_3**
   i.   Small lesions by transurethral resection or diathermy
   ii. Larger lesions by:
      a.   Transurethral resection
      b.   Open transvesical excision
      c.   Less commonly partial cystectomy. This is less popular now and is used mainly for adenocarcinoma
   iii. All patients should be followed up with repeated cystoscopy to treat such recurrences as may occur

2. **Large, deep or extensive lesions by combinations of surgery, radiotherapy and chemotherapy**

Surgery
  i.   Partial cystectomy, see above
  ii. Total cystectomy with urinary diversion (*see* Urinary diversion p. 91). Very widespread multiple lesions may require extensive surgery up to nephro-uretero-cysto-prostato-urethrectomy
  iii. Occasionally complete pelvic clearance is indicated

Chemotherapy
  i.   Local with instillation of surface acting agents, e.g. 'thiotepa', 'epodyl'. Some absorption may occur and lead to bone marrow depression

Riddle, P.R. & Wallace, D.M. (1971) Intracavitary chemotherapy for multiple non-invasive bladder tumours. *British Journal of Urology,* **43**, 181-184.

  ii. Systemic chemotherapy with various agents

Radiotherapy
  i.   Local implantation with radon, gold or tantalum Suitable for tumours up to 3 cm diameter, over that size too much necrosis occurs in the centre
  ii. Local infusion of colloidal gold, sodium or bromine salts

Wallace, D.M. (1971) Intracavitary radiation for multiple non-infiltrating bladder tumours. *British Journal of Urology,* **43**, 177-180.

  iii. External irradiation by supervoltage, cobalt or accelerator units

Other techniques
  a.   Hydrostatic pressure technique of Helmstein Used for extensive T$_1$ tumours and to control haemorrhage in advanced inoperable tumours

Glashan, R.W. (1975) A critical review of the management of bladder neoplasia using a modified form of Helmstein's pressure therapy. *British Journal of Urology,* **47**, 57-66.
Hammonds, J.C., Williams, J.C. & Fox, M. (1974) The control of severe bleeding from the bladder by intravesical hyperbaric therapy. *British Journal of Urology,* **46**, 309-312.
Helmstein, K. (1972) Treatment of bladder carcinoma by a hydrostatic pressure technique. *British Journal of Urology,* **44**, 434-450.

  b.   Immunotherapy with sensitised pig lymphocytes.

Fenely, R.C.L., Eckert, H., Riddell, A.G., Symes, M.O. & Tribe, C.R. (1974) The treatment of advanced bladder cancer with sensitized pig lymphocytes. *British Journal of Surgery,* **61**, 825-827.

FURTHER READING
Miller, A. & Mitchell, J.P. (1969) The Bristol Bladder Tumour Registry. *British Journal of Urology,* **41**, Supplement.
Wallace, D.M. (1972) Urothelial neoplasia—causes, assessment and treatment. *Annals of the Royal College of Surgeons of England,* **51**, 91-102.

Methods of urinary diversion

May be classified as follows:
  Temporary or permanent
  Intubated or non-intubated
  Supravesical or vesical

1. NEPHROSTOMY

  i. Lower pole (inferior calyx) nephrostomy by Malecot or de Pezzor catheters

  ii. Loop nephrostomy with Silastic catheter is especially useful in the following situations:
    a. Small intrarenal pelvis
    b. When nephrostomy drainage is likely to be prolonged as in severe inflammation, stricture or stenosis at ureteropelvic junction
    c. Where it is essential that the nephrostomy tube can't fall out as in a pyonephrosis of an obstructed solitary kidney

Hawtrey, E.C., Boatman, D.L., Brown, R.G. & Schmidt, J.D. (1974) Clinical experience with loop nephrostomy for urinary diversion. *Journal of Urology*, **112**, 36-41.

Tressidder, G.C. (1957) Nephrostomy. *British Journal of Urology*, **29**, 130-134.

2. LOOP CUTANEOUS URETEROSTOMY

  i. Provides temporary diversion usually in neonates or infants with advanced hydro-ureter and hydronephrosis caused by lower urinary tract obstruction (usually posterior urethral valves). These children have severe electrolyte imbalance and uraemia as a result of advanced renal impairment

  ii. The loop should be constructed from the dilated and tortuous ureter as close as possible to the ureteropelvic junction to provide effective decompression of obstructed kidneys

  iii. Loop ureterostomy should not be closed (by excision of loop and re-anastomosis of ureter over T-tube ureterostomy *in situ*) before optimal anatomical and functional recovery of dilated upper tracts

3.   END CUTANEOUS URETEROSTOMY

Rarely indicated except as a swift diversion in sick children with congenital defect (spina bifida, ectopia vesica, sacral agensis) where the lower urinary tract will never be functional. Skin flaps are used to construct a spout and to prevent stomal stenosis. If the general condition improves, can be converted to conduit diversion in later childhood.

4.   URETEROSTOMY *IN SITU*

i.   Intubation of an unmobilised ureter. Often a simpler alternative to nephrostomy

ii.   May be used as an adjunct to conservative surgical procedures on the upper urinary tract or to relieve the acute anuria of ureteric obstruction

5.   SUPRAPUBIC CYSTOSTOMY

i.   Bladder neck obstruction
ii.   Urethral trauma
iii.   Urethral stricture

6.   URETEROSIGMOIDOSTOMY

i.   Was the method of choice for urinary diversion before the introduction of conduits

ii.   The disadvantages were:
a.   Ascending infection and chronic pyelonephritis
b.   Hyperchloraemic acidosis. Hypokalaemia. Controlled by low salt diet, high fluid intake, regular alkali ingestion, frequent bowel evacuation and night time use of rectal tube
c.   Incontinence of liquid stool when anal sphincter tone was inadequate

iii.   In about 60% of patients this procedure is compatible with low morbidity and long term survival. The added convenience of continence and freedom from stoma care and appliance management are obvious

iv.   Rapid deterioration of the upper urinary tract was found to correlate with a high intracolonic pressure and, in this group of patients, sigmoid-myotomy has been performed synchronously to lower colonic pressure

Jacobs, A. (1967) A review of long-term results of uretero-colic anastomosis. *British Journal of Urology,* **39,** 670-675.
Daniel, O. & Ram, R.S. (1965) The value of sigmoid-myotomy in reducing bowel pressure and thus averting renal damage following ureterocolic anastomosis. *British Journal of Urology,* **37,** 654-659.

7. URETERO-URETEROSTOMY

i. Indicated for condition involving the distal ureter with a normal contralateral ureter. An alternative to:
   a. Psoas-hitch and ureteric reimplantation
   b. Bladder flap (Boari) ureteroplasty
ii. Contra-indicated where ureteric obstruction is due to malignant disease or irradiation ureteric stricture

8. ILEAL CONDUIT

The preferred method of permanent urinary diversion in adults and children. The peristaltic activity of ileum is greater than that of colon ensuring rapid emptying of conduit and prevention of urine stasis, bacterial overgrowth and retrograde urinary infection. Reflux preventing mechanisms (at uretero-ileal anastomosis) are not attempted, being necessary in reservoirs not conduits. In children with spina bifida there is no agreement as to the best time for urinary diversion.

The stoma should be constructed away from bony prominences, skin creases and scars. Complications include stenosis at uretero-ileal anastomosis, stomal stenosis, skin excoriation, conduit calculus formation and, rarely, adenocarcinoma of ileal conduit.

Johnston, J.H. (1974) Pyelo-colonic diversion in children. *British Journal of Urology,* **46**, 169-172.

Scott, J.E.S. (1973) Urinary diversion in children. *Archives of Disease in Childhood,* **48**, 199-206.

Wallace, D.M. (1966) Ureteric diversion using a conduit: a simplified technique. *British Journal of Urology,* **38**, 522-527.

Wallace, D.M. (1970) Uretero-ileostomy. *British Journal of Urology,* **42**, 529-534.

9. COLON CONDUIT

i. Because of the thicker wall of the colon, ureters may be anastomosed in an anti-reflux fashion (Leadbetter and Clarke, 1955) Theoretically this should reduce the incidence of post-operative pyelonephritis
ii. Stomal stenosis may occur with the ileal or colonic conduit. Because of the greater diameter of the colon and the wider stoma, the incidence of stomal stenosis may be reduced
iii. The colon conduit is probably free from electrolyte disturbance
iv. Following pelvic exenteration (persistent or recurrent neoplasia of cervix, endometrium or vagina after irradiation) a colon conduit has the advantage of avoiding an intestinal anastomosis

v.   In spina bifida (the commonest indication for urinary diversion in children) chronic constipation may make adequate colonic preparation difficult

Leadbetter, W.F. & Clarke, B.G. (1955) Five years' experience with uretero-enterostomy by the 'combined' technique. *Journal of Urology,* **73**, 67-82.
Mogg, R.A. & Syme, R.R.A. (1969) The results of urinary diversion using the colon conduit. *British Journal of Urology,* **41**, 434-447.

10. RECTAL BLADDER

Ureters transplanted to a rectal bladder with terminal sigmoid colostomy. No intestinal anastomosis involved. Almost the whole length of both ureters must be preserved for anastomosis without tension whereas conduit diversion is at the pelvic brim.

i.   Primary rectal bladder
ii.   Secondary rectal bladder. If, following uretero-sigmoidostomy, there is progressive upper tract damage, a terminal colostomy can be constructed

Hanley, H.G. (1967) The rectal bladder. *British Journal of Urology,* **39**, 693-695.

Trauma to the urinary tract

MECHANISMS

1. *Deceleration:* especially affects kidney and upper tract
2. *Direct injury*
   i. To kidney
   ii. To a full bladder predisposing it to rupture
   iii. To the perineal urethra
3. *Penetrating injury*
   i. From outside the body to any part of the urinary tract
   ii. Penetration of the lower urinary tract by a pelvic fracture
4. *Indirect trauma:* disruption of the symphysis leading to urethral injury
5. *Iatrogenic injury*
   i. To ureter during pelvic dissection or laparoscopy
   ii. To bladder during pelvic surgery or during transurethral procedures

GENERAL MANAGEMENT

1. Suspicion of the possibility in suitable trauma
2. Await micturition
3. Inspect and test urine for blood
4. Appropriate radiology; intravenous urography, cystography or urethrography, arteriography. See below
5. Bed rest until macroscopic haematuria ceases
6. Blood transfusion and intravenous fluids as necessary
7. Catheter only if essential; if lower tract injury then suprapubic cystostomy
8. Some use routine antibiotics

MANAGEMENT AT OPERATION FOR OTHER REASONS

1. Perinephric haematoma only needs exploration if expanding
2. Urine in the peritoneum. Repair the tear. Drain the bladder/perinephric space
3. Divided ureter—as below

RADIOLOGY

All patients with suspected renal trauma should have an intravenous urogram

Abnormalities demonstrated on urogram:
1. Mild injury; no abnormality
2. Moderate injury: delayed opacification, filling defects due to blood clot in the collecting system, spastic calyces, large or blurred kidney outline, extravasation of urine
3. Severe injury; some or all of the collecting system is not visible or there may be total non-opacification
4. Extravasation in the lower tract may be demonstrated

Indications for arteriography:
1. Expanding loin haematoma
2. Signs of severe injury on intravenous urography
3. Macroscopic haematuria lasting over 7 days
4. Later for hypertension or suspected arteriovenous fistula

Findings on arteriography:
1. Non-filling of all or part of the renal vasculature due to major vessel damage
2. Cortical lacerations
3. Later arteriogram may show cortical atrophy or areas of ischaemia

Radioactive hippuran scan may be an alternative method of demonstrating absent blood flow in a kidney

Cystography is rarely of value since most bladder injuries may be diagnosed clinically. Since it requires catheterisation it may itself increase damage

Urethrography is used by some in the early management of urethral trauma but more tend to use it later to demonstrate complex strictures

KIDNEY
1. Damage to the kidney rarely needs surgery and may be managed conservatively. However progressive hypovolaemic shock with an expanding loin haematoma indicates major kidney damage and may need nephrectomy. These patients may not be fit for radiological investigation or need intervention before that can be arranged
2. Major vessel damage can occasionally be repaired if only the intima is damaged
3. Segmental injury may be managed by partial nephrectomy
4. Later surgery may be required for areas of local ischaemia or for secondary hydronephrosis

URETER

1. Damage by cutting at operation can usually be repaired primarily
2. Damage by diathermy may devitalise a segment which needs excising
3. Damage by a penetrating missile may devitalise a segment the size of which can be difficult to determine at primary operation and may need a secondary procedure following temporary diversion by nephrostomy
4. Segment loss at the upper end will require urinary diversion (see p. 89)
5. Segment loss at the lower end may be treated by reimplantation if necessary supplemented by a bladder flap or bladder hitch to the psoas

BLADDER

1. Intraperitoneal or extraperitoneal urine leak is not a serious problem for 24 to 48 hours and hence suspected injuries can be safely observed for a period
2. Intraperitoneal rupture may be repaired and drained with a urethral catheter
3. Extraperitoneal rupture may be repaired and drained suprapubically. The retropubic space is also drained. Spontaneous micturition is awaited or alternatively the urethra may be inspected endoscopically at about two weeks

URETHRA

Many urethral injuries are incomplete and may be rendered complete by ill advised instrumentation
Diagnosis on:
1. Mechanism of injury
2. Blood at external urinary meatus
3. Failure to pass urine
4. Palpable bladder
Regimes of treatment:
1. Early suprapubic catheter or cystostomy; or await micturition and insert suprapubic catheter if this does not occur
    At about two weeks urethroscopy or urethrography
    Formal repair over a catheter
2. Early urethroscopy or urethrography
    Partial tear—suprapubic catheter
    Complete tear—formal repair over catheter, traction applied by stitch through prostate to thigh. Traction applied through a catheter is unreliable and liable to lead to necrosis

3.   Tear associated with fracture or disruption of the symphysis pubis; explore suprapubically and repair over a fenestrated catheter

FURTHER READING

Mitchell, J.P. (1971) Trauma to the urinary tract. *British Medical Journal*, ii, 567-573.

Pryor, J.P. & Williams, J.P. (1975) A study of 137 cases of renal trauma. *British Journal of Urology*, **47**, 45-49.

Turner Warwick, R. (1973) Observations on the treatment of traumatic urethral injuries and the value of the fenestrated catheter. *British Journal of Surgery*, **60**, 775-781.

Renal transplantation

TRANSPLANTATION ANTIGENS
Histocompatibility antigens are genetically determined and specific to one individual and not to the organ transplanted. In man, the major histocompatability antigens are present on the surface of most cell types in the body and are known as human leucocyte associated antigens (HL-A antigens). The HL-A system in man is responsible for graft versus host reaction and delayed hypersensitivity.

HL-A system
1. Every human carries 4 out of a possible 30 antigens; 2 inherited from each parent resulting in up to 8,000 phenotypes in the population
2. Each parent and child, therefore, will have 2 HL-A antigens in common
3. Non-identical siblings have:
   1:4 chance of sharing all 4 antigens
   2:4 chance of sharing 2 antigens
   1:4 chance of not sharing any histocompatability antigens

DONOR SELECTION
1. ABO blood group compatibility is absolutely essential
2. HL-A compatability
   i. Excellent results are achieved (assessed by graft survival and function) if all 4 HL-A antigens are compatible in donor and recipient. This situation occurs in identical twins but non-identical siblings have a 1:4 chance of inheriting the same HL-A antigens. Many authors believe that this is the only situation where HL-A typing is of any value
   ii. A difference of one or more HL-A antigens gives uniformly poorer results whether the donor and recipient are related or unrelated. The graft prognosis seems to be unaffected by the number of HL-A incompatibilities
3. Mixed lymphocyte culture
When donor and recipient lymphocytes are cultured together, the percentage of cells transforming to blast cells is inversely proportional to tissue compatibility and graft prognosis. Since the results of mixed lymphocyte culture are read at about one week, this superior test is unsuitable for cadaver kidney transplantation

PRESERVATION OF CADAVER KIDNEY

1. Normothermic renal ischaemia exceeding 70 to 90 minutes results in irreversible tubular or cortical damage
2. A common practice is to perfuse the kidney briefly with a high molecular weight dextran until the kidney becomes pale, and then with a buffered sugar solution at $4^{\circ}C$. If the kidney is then preserved on ice (surface cooling) a complete recovery of function can follow a total ischaemic time of 12 hours
3. In vitro pulsatile perfusion with either oxygenated blood, at $37^{\circ}C$, or oxygen-saturated macromolecules (albumin, dextran, fluorocarbons) may prolong the total ischaemia time without the risk of tubular or cortical necrosis
4. The warm ischaemia time is necessarily prolonged in the U.K. by the legal requirement that heart and respiratory function must cease before the cadaver kidney is removed

TECHNIQUE OF TRANSPLANTATION

The right iliac fossa is the most favourable site for transplantation for the following reasons:

   i. Technically simpler than the low lumbar position or the normal anatomical position
   ii. The graft is superficial making biopsy and assessment of change in volume easier
   iii. Further surgery for any complication of renal transplantation is easier at this site
   iv. Preferable to LIF where the pelvic mesocolon must be reflected in preparing the graft bed. Some authors prefer to transplant the left kidney to LIF. The RIF is suitable if the left kidney is rotated so that its anterior surface lies posteriorly

1. Oblique muscle cutting incision. Extraperitoneal approach to RIF and the vessels at the pelvic brim
2. The renal vein is anastomosed end-to-side with the common iliac vein
3. The renal artery is anastomosed end-to-end with the internal iliac artery
4. The ureter is anastomosed either to the recipient ureter making synchronous ipsilateral nephrectomy necessary, or to the recipient bladder by a reflux-preventing mechanism

COMPLICATIONS OF RENAL TRANSPLANTATION

1. Acute tubular necrosis
  i. Rarely seen with a living donor kidney because the total ischaemia time can be reduced to a minimum
  ii. Usually seen in the cadaver kidney when the total ischaemia time is prolonged or where the donor was hypotensive before death
  iii. Haemodialysis may be necessary during the anuric phase
  iv. During the diuretic phase when urine is hyperosmolar, dehydration hyponatraemia and hypokalaemia can occur unless i.v. fluids are titrated against urinary volume and measured electrolyte loss

2. Acute rejection
  i. Fever and swelling of the transplanted kidney
  ii. A sudden fall in urinary volume with proteinuria and the appearance of lymphocytes in the urine
  iii. A fall in creatinine and urea clearance with a rise in blood levels. A low urinary sodium
  iv. Fibrin deposition in the transplanted kidney detected by [125]Fibrinogen
  v. Renal biopsy shows perivascular lymphocyte infiltration and interstitial oedema
  vi. May respond to adding Actinomycin C to the immunosuppressive regime

3. Chronic rejection
  Can be detected by biopsy long before deterioration in renal function develops. Foci of lymphocyte aggregation are seen affecting predominantly either the glomerulus, interstitial tissues or arterioles. Gradually proteinuria, hypertension and renal failure develop

4. Stricture or fistula at ureteric anastomosis
  i. Due to inadequate blood supply of the donor ureter and to poor healing in uraemic patients on immunosuppressive therapy
  ii. Less common with uretero-ureterostomy (than ureterocystostomy) because a shorter length of donor ureter is required
  iii. A fistula may be associated with the cystostomy necessary for ureterocystostomy

5. Renal artery thrombosis or stenosis

6. **Urinary tract infection is encouraged by:**
   i. The increased susceptibility to infection of uraemic patients on immunosuppressive therapy
   ii. A ureteric catheter used to splint the uretero-ureterostomy (and brought to the surface either trans-urethrally or by suprapubic cystostomy)
   iii. A urethral catheter necessary to protect a cystostomy

7. **Tertiary hyperparathyroidism**

COMPLICATIONS OF IMMUNOSUPPRESSION

1. **Steroids**
   i. Impaired wound healing
   ii. Increased susceptibility to infections including herpes simplex, herpes zoster, viral hepatitis and mycoses
   iii. Gastrointestinal bleeding and pancreatitis
   iv. Avascular bone necrosis. Osteoporosis
   v. Cushing's syndrome
   vi. Cataract
   vii. Diabetes
   vii. Psychosis

2. **Antimetabolites**
   Usually Azathioprine but occasionally 6-Mercaptopurine or Methotrexate
   i. Hepatotoxicity
   ii. Marrow depression
   iii. Oncogenicity (lymphoma)

3. **Antilymphocyte serum**
   (Serum from horses immunised with human thoracic duct lymphocytes or thymus. Antibodies to red cells, platelets and fibrinogen are adsorbed by contact with washed red cells, platelets and plasma)
   i. Inflammation and pain at injection site
   ii. Thrombocytopenia. Antiplatelet antibodies are difficult to remove by adsorption and it is difficult to prevent platelet contamination of lymphocytes used for horse immunisation
   iii. Allergy to foreign protein. Urticaria, serum sickness and anaphylaxis
   iv. Oncogenicity (lymphoma)

FURTHER READING
Hall, C.L. *et al.* (1976) Results of 250 consecutive cadaver kidney transplants. *British Medical Journal*, i, 547-550.
Woodruff, M.F.A. *et al.* (1976) Long survival after renal transplantation in man. *British Journal of Surgery*, **63**, 85-101.

Implants, non-biological materials

REQUIREMENTS
1. Physical properties suitable for the task
   i. Tensile strength—sutures, bone plates
   ii. Load bearing strength—total hip replacement
   iii. Flexibility—tendons, breast prosthesis, catheters
   iv. Compatible metals to avoid electrolytic corrosion
   v. Wear resistance for moving implants
2. Not modified by tissues
   i. Loss of flexibility of elastomers
   ii. Corrosion of metals
3. Acceptable biocompatibility
   i. Not promoting inflammatory reaction
   ii. Not releasing toxic chemicals. (Catalysts and other additives)
   iii. Not carcinogenic—some metal microparticles are carcinogenic in animals
   iv. Not antigenic
   v. Not allergenic
4. Capable of construction to patterns required
5. Capable of sterilisation

USES
1. Repair
2. Reconstruction
3. Replacement
4. Support

PROBLEMS AND COMPLICATIONS
1. Limited life span of materials
2. Variable fixation to tissues
3. Infection, direct and haematogenous
4. Adsorption of chemicals. Many plastics adsorb chemicals on contact with skin and liquid/gas sterilising agents
5. Variable and limited physical properties
   i. Bone plates will not bear weight
   ii. Some sponges become hard
   iii. Catheters may become hard
6. Need for revision with growth
   i. Arthroplasties in Still's disease
   ii. Distal catheter of Spitz Holter valve

MATERIALS

Metals

1. *Stainless steels*
   Bone plates and screws
   Arthroplasties
2. *Chrome-cobalt alloys*
   Bone plates and screws
   Arthroplasties
   (Cast alloys have low torsional strength)
3. *Tantalum. Titanium*
   Bone plates and screws
   Mandibles
   Mesh: coarse—acetabulum false floor
             fine—hernia repair

Textiles

1. *Dacron', 'terylene'*
   i.   Woven tubes
       Small interstices
       Small blood loss
       Poor penetration by fibrous tissue
       Poor fixation of pseudo-intima
       Used for large vessel replacement
       Knitted tubes
        Large interstices, therefore pre-clotting required
        Good fibrous tissue penetration
        Therefore good adherence of pseudo-intima
        More suitable for small vessel replacement
   ii. Sheets and felts for attachments
       Heart valves
       Breast prostheses
   iii. Spun
       Sutures, esp. vascular—low drag
2. *Nylon*
   i.   Sheets—for hernia repair
   ii. Extruded—monofilament sutures
   iii. Braided—sutures
3. *'Teflon', 'fluon'*
   Similar uses to 'Dacron'

Plastics
1. *Teflon*
   Stapes implants
2. *Polyethylene*
   i.   Low density—facial implants
   ii. High density—self-lubricating properties
        Joint replacement
3. *Polymethylmethacrylate*
   i.   'Cold-polymerising'—used as bone cement
   ii. Occasionally as solid implant—cranioplasty
4. *Polyurethane*
   Sponge used in rectal prolapse

Elastomers
Silicone rubbers used for 'rubbery' implants
Dimethyl siloxane 'Silastic'
1. *Prefashioned*
   i.   'Spacers' in arthroplasty of small joints
   ii. Replacement of small bones
   iii. Rods to encourage epithelial 'sheath' formation prior
        to tendon transplant
   iv. Encasing fluids in breast prosthesis
2. *Fashioned in situ*
   i.   Custom made prostheses—chin implants
   ii. Sheets to prevent adhesion formation, e.g. after
        tenolysis

Fluids
Silicones
1. Injectable augmentation of tissues
2. Lubrication of joints

Composite examples
1. *Heart valves*
   i.   Chrome cobalt cage
   ii. Silicone rubber ball
   iii. Dacron cover
2. *Breasts*
   i.   Silicone fluid
   ii. Silicone rubber case
   iii. Dacron felt fixation
3. *Joints*
   i.   High density polyethylene (acetabulum, tibial
        condyles)
   ii. Chrome cobalt/steel (head of femur, femoral
        condyles)

Burns

TYPE OF BURN

Thermal
　　May be further subdivided depending on exact mechanism,
　　e.g. wet/dry, flash or flame contact, direct contact with
　　burning fluids
Electrical
　　High voltage burns are complicated by deep necrosis of
　　tissues between entry and exit
Chemical
　　May continue to progress in depth and severity if the
　　causative chemical is not completely removed
Radiation
　　May be much more extensive than superficial appearances
　　suggest

DEPTH OF BURN

For treatment differentiation three categories only are needed:
Superficial
　　Epidermis and superficial dermis only
Deep dermal
　　Preserving a few of the deepest dermal epithelial
　　components, e.g. sweat duct epithelium
Deep
　　No dermal epithelium left

DIAGNOSIS OF DEPTH

　　Appearance may be very deceptive with different
　　mechanisms
Jackson, D.M. (1970) In search of an acceptable burn classification. *British
Journal of Plastic Surgery*, **23**, 219-226.
　　Pin-prick sensation is lost in deep burns and certain chemical
　　burns, e.g. phenol
　　Thermography reveals areas where the skin plexus of vessels
　　has been destroyed or has no flow due to intravascular
　　coagulation

DIAGNOSIS OF AREA

　　The 'Rule of Nines' is very useful in adults but may be very
　　inaccurate in children especially up to one year where the
　　head and neck amount to 20% of body surface area

PROGNOSIS

Mortality rate increases with age. As a rough guide in most cases where the age plus the percentage area is over 100 the chances of survival are very poor.

MANAGEMENT

1. **Primary treatment**
   i. Remove the burning agent
   ii. Pain relief
   iii. Fluid replacement for superficial burns and small areas of deep burn
      a. Crystalloid solution
      b. High molecular weight dextrans
      c. Plasma
      d. Plasma protein fraction
      Simple formula for fluid replacement is that of:
      120mls/1% burn (up to 6 litres) in 48 h
      This is given in aliquots of:
         half in first 8 h
         quarter in next 16 h
         quarter in final 24 h
         (Evans, 1975)
      In children the replacement regime needs to be more closely related to their surface area
      This is a rough guide and fluid replacement should be monitored against:
      a. repeated haematocrit
      b. observation of urine output which should be over 25 ml per hour
      c. measurement of serum electrolytes and osmolality
      d. blood gas measurement
      e. central venous pressure
      Patients with over 10% deep burn also need blood replacement, approximately one percent of the blood volume being replaced per ten percent of burn
   iv. Encircling burns constrict and exert a tourniquet effect on limbs and restrict respiration when involving the chest wall. These should be divided to their full depth as part of the primary treatment initiated in the Accident Department

2. **Secondary treatment** (after the first 48 h)
    General care of the patient is aimed at maintaining a good general state in this highly catabolic condition. This is achieved by maintaining the haemoglobin and the level of nutrition; if necessary by parenteral feeding and vitamin supplements
    Some advocate administration of zinc salts

3. **Tertiary treatment**
    General rehabilitation including job placement
    Further reconstructive surgery to scars—often delayed by 18 months

LOCAL MANAGEMENT OF BURN

Aims of local care of the burn:
  i.   Prevent further tissue loss
  ii. Aid rapid healing with minimal infection, minimal scar and minimal secondary deformity

1. **Exposure techniques**
    i.   On an open bed with sterile linen changed frequently
    ii. On sterilised polyurethane foam
    iii. By 'levitation' on:
        a. An air-loss type of bed
        b. An air fluidised bed
        c. A water bed
    iv. Prevent infection by:
        a. Laminar air flow rooms
        b. Keeping exposed surface dry
        c. Trying to prevent cracks
        d. Applying antiseptics to flexures and face

2. **Dressing techniques**
    i.   Dressings applied in theatre conditions
    ii. Prevent infection by:
        a. Silver nitrate 0.5% soaks—must keep moist
        b. Sulphamylon cream
        c. Silver sulphadiazine cream—effective but expensive

3. **Use of heterograft**
    i.   Very convenient material
    ii. Large sheets are readily prepared and applied
    iii. Must be removed and replaced with autograft or fresh heterograft by 10 days since it tends to become incorporated and provoke an antibody response creating more extensive scarring

4. **Early grafting techniques**
   i.   Small local deep dermal or deep burn
         Excision and suture or primary graft
   ii.   Early excision and grafting
         Performed at 48 h. Major procedure that can be
         performed on up to 15% burn. Priorities are face, neck,
         hands, flexures
         Excised with knife or carbon dioxide laser
         Grafted with autograft, homograft, or heterograft
   iii. Tangential grafting
         Especially useful for deep dermal burns
         Burnt area is excised using a skin-graft knife until
         healthy tissue is reached
         Grafted as above

5. **Later grafting**
   Performed after the fourteenth day when the eschar is
   separating and when the final thickness of the burn has been
   definitely established
   The eschar is excised and then grafted as above
   Autograft may be 'extended' to cover a larger area by a
   number of methods such as strip grafting, converting the split
   skin to an extendible mesh

FURTHER READING
Evans, A.J. (1975) The modern treatment of burns. *British Journal of Hospital Medicine*, **13**, 287-298.
Sanders, R. (1974) The burnt patient: a general view. *British Medical Journal*, iii, 460-463.

Skin flaps and transfers

Flaps and transfers are used to move full thickness skin from one site to another

TRADITIONAL METHODS
Free graft
Advantage: One stage procedure
Disadvantage: Unreliable take
Suitable for small areas only

Tube pedicle

Advantage: Can be swung anywhere
Disadvantage: Limited length relative to width
Protracted multiple surgery with possibility of loss or shortening of the pedicle at each stage
Prolonged immobilisation

Local rotation flaps
Advantage: One stage procedure
Uses skin of same or similar quality to that of the defect
Disadvantage: Usually only possible once
Needs a very long base which may be limited by local anatomy
Easy for it not to fit if not meticulously planned.

Cross transfers (e.g. cross-finger, cross-leg)
Advantage: Similar skin
Usually can be simply planned with a template
Disadvantage: Requires immobilisation of the healthy limb or digit

NEWER TECHNIQUES

Vascular pedicle flap
This is a flap based on an axial artery, e.g. temporal artery, branch of internal mammary, neuro-vascular island pedicle in the fingers
Advantage: Large areas of skin may be obtained
There may be a small base for a long flap
The flap survives well

Free vascular flap
An area of skin is entirely detached with its supplying vessel(s)
which are reanastomosed to vessels in the recipient area

Advantage:	Single stage procedure
	Large areas of skin may be moved
Disadvantage:	Requires skilled microvascular surgery using
	an operating microscope
	The flap is very thick

FURTHER READING
Cobbett, J.R. (1975) Microvascular surgery. *British Journal of Hospital Medicine,* **13**, 311-318.

Spina bifida

Careful individual assessment of all cases at birth, but with rare exceptions (e.g. thoraco-lumbar lesions with little paralysis)
Active treatment only in the absence of the following *adverse prognostic criteria*
1. Thoraco-lumbar myelomeningocele
2. Severe paraplegia. (Weak hip flexors only)
3. Congenital hydrocephalus
   Head circumference above 90th percentile corrected for birth weight
   Bulging anterior fontanelle and wide skull sutures
4. Kyphosis
5. Presence of other severe congenital defects or birth trauma

On these criteria one third of patients are treated. The remaining two thirds are fed on demand, but no antibiotics should be prescribed, no resuscitation undertaken and no painful investigations performed. The parents should not be encouraged to take the baby home. In most series these severely handicapped babies die in the first months of life.
Patients with *adverse prognostic criteria* who are actively treated from birth:
1. Are likely to die in infancy from ventriculitis and the effects of associated congenital defects
2. Are likely to have hydrocephalus and a low I.Q.
3. Are likely to develop hydronephrosis, chronic pyelonephritis, hypertension and renal failure
4. Will have more hospital admissions for shunt, urinary and orthopaedic procedures
5. Are likely to be chair bound
6. Are likely to have severe scoliosis, kyphosis, osteoporosis and pathological fractures
7. Are likely to have sacral, perineal and leg anaesthesia with trophic ulceration
8. Are likely to require permanent care

Selected patients should be treated vigorously with special reference to:
1. Early closure of myelomeningocele
2. Recognition and treatment of hydrocephalus
3. Preservation of renal function
4. Timely orthopaedic intervention

EARLY CLOSURE OF MYELOMENINGOCELE

To ensure against meningitis, ventriculitis and further deterioration of limb and pelvic visceral innervation
Surgical procedure
1. A thin membrane which covers the neural plaque is removed
2. The neural plaque is exposed centrally and dura is seen at the margin of the defect attached to skin
3. Dura and skin are separated. The dura is mobilised circumferentially and the dural tube reconstituted. In the lumbar region this repair can be reinforced by transposed flaps of lumbar fascia
4. Skin flaps are mobilised into the flanks to achieve skin closure without tension

Complications
1. Meningitis.
    Especially if closure is undertaken after 24 hours from birth
2. Skin dehiscence
    i.   Suture line tension because of inadequate skin flap mobilisation
    ii.   Imperfect haemostasis and the collection of blood clots beneath flaps
    iii. CSF leak from reconstituted dural tube, especially if CSF pressure is rising.
3. Wound infection from faecal stream

RECOGNITION AND TREATMENT OF HYDROCEPHALUS

Indications for treatment of hydrocephalus
1. Rapid increase in occipito-frontal circumference of a normal-sized head
2. Wide skull sutures, especially occipito-parietal suture
3. CSF pressure (ventriculostomy) greater than 300mm CSF
4. Air ventriculography:
    i. Cerebral thickness of 35mm or more is not associated with progressive hydrocephalus
    ii. Cerebral thickness of 25 to 35mm may not indicate progressive disease especially if CSF pressure is less than 300mm of CSF
    iii. Cerebral thickness less than 25mm is usually, but not necessarily, an indication of progressive hydrocephalus

Complications of ventricular drainage
(The distal catheter of ventricular shunt system may be drained either into the right atrium or peritoneal cavity.)
1. Proximal catheter block by choroid plexus
2. Distal catheter block:
    i. By retraction of catheter with growth into a thrombosed vein
    ii. By peritoneal loculation
3. Colonisation of valve (usually by a coagulase -ve *staph. albus*)
    i. Septicaemia (with atrial drainage)
    ii. Peritonitis (with peritoneal drainage)
4. Pulmonary hypertension. The result of recurrent microembolisation from catheter tip
5. 'Shunt nephritis'. Haematuria and progressive renal damage associated with a colonised valve

Definite indications should exist before ventricular drainage is performed, because in one series, shunt complications cause a mortality of 20% over 8 years

PRESERVATION OF RENAL FUNCTION

Three patterns of abnormality may exist as defined by IVP and cysto-urethrography

1. Normal or hyperactive detrusor contractions without bladder neck obstruction. Manual expression unnecessary because dribbling is continuous and bladder emptying is complete
2. Hypotonic detrusor without bladder neck obstruction. Manual expression is indicated
3. Normal detrusor activity with bladder neck obstruction. Should be treated initially by urethral dilation in females and sphincterotomy in males

Indications for urinary diversion

1. Recurrent episodes of urinary tract infection especially if there is evidence of upper tract damage
2. Bladder neck obstruction inadequately controlled by urethral dilation or sphincterotomy, especially if there is evidence of developing hydro-ureter or hydronephrosis
3. When it is obvious that no continence will develop, especially as school age approaches, when continence in a child mobile on crutches and/or calipers may mean attending a normal school rather than one for the physically handicapped

Methods of urinary diversion

1. Ileal conduit. An adequate spout and expert stoma supervision will prevent skin contamination
2. Colon conduit
   i. May be difficult to empty the colon pre-operatively in these chronically constipated children
   ii. Selective electrolyte reabsorption and hyperchloraemic acidosis may result, especially if there is any deterioration of renal function and consequent loss of compensating capacity
3. Loop or end cutaneous ureterostomy. May be indicated as a temporary or permanent procedure in sick children. It has the advantages of being a swifter procedure without the risk of anastomotic complications

See Urinary diversion, p. 89

ORTHOPAEDIC MANAGEMENT

Neonatal deformity is dependent on
 The level of paralysis
 The intra-uterine posture
Later development of deformity is dependent on
 Degree of maintained mobility in the joints
 Action of unopposed muscles—dependent on the level of
 paralysis
 Effects of trauma, iatrogenic and otherwise
Patients may be divided into three broad groups
 i. Paralysis below T12/L1. Flaccid paraplegia with, at
   most, a very weak psoas
 ii. Paralysis below L3. Strong hip flexors and adductors,
   may have knee extension depending on extent of
   involvement of L3. Mainly hip problems
 iii. Paralysis below L5. Main problems are below the knee
Principles of management
 Deformity from total paralysis may usually be corrected and
 maintained by passive stretching and splinting
 Deformity from partial paralysis is maintained by unopposed
 muscle action and therefore needs muscle rebalancing
 Correction required distally may be modified by results of
 treatment of proximal deformity

Hip
 Dislocation. Reduction may be obtained by the usual methods
 but usually requires surgery to rebalance the muscles
 Deformity. Usually flexion and adduction. Will need surgery to
 rebalance the muscles
 Muscle rebalancing.
 i. Weak flexors and adductors (up to M.R.C. grade 3)
   probably just need division of the adductor origin and
   psoas insertion. Fixed deformity may require more
   extensive release and varus osteotomy
 ii. With powerful flexors and adductors (grades of 4+ or 5) a
   more formal rebalancing with iliopsoas transfer to an
   insertion on the greater trochanter via the ilium may be
   necessary

Mustard, W.T. (1959) A follow-up study of iliopsoas transfer for hip instability. *Journal of Bone and Joint Surgery,* **41B**, 289-298.
Sharrard, W.J.W. (1964) Posterior iliopsoas transplantation in the treatment of paralytic dislocation of the hip. *Journal of Bone and Joint Surgery,* **46B**, 426-444.

Knee

Flexion deformity may often be corrected passively. If division of hamstrings is required posterior capsulotomy should be avoided unless essential since it may lead to later recurvatum

If the knee extensors are powerful quadriceps lengthening may be required

Varus or valgus can be corrected by osteotomy

Foot

Equinovarus or calcaneovalgus can be corrected by routine methods. Soft tissue release is frequently needed. Bizarre or very stiff deformities may be helped by astragalectomy

Spine

Lordosis. Usually secondary to hip deformity and resolves when the hip is corrected. If very stiff it may require surgery

Kyphosis. May be very acutely angled preventing upright posture and may greatly impede access to the abdomen, e.g. for urinary diversion. Spinal osteotomy and fusion may be performed but frequently at the cost of total loss of function below that level.

Scoliosis. May be treated as other scolioses, often suitable for correction by the anterior route. Low scoliosis with fixed pelvic obliquity can be corrected by spinal osteotomy but it is often easier to accept the deformity, stabilise the hip and shorten the opposite leg.

Trauma

Skin ulceration is a problem especially for the mobile patient as in any other paraparetic patient

Fracture of the porotic bones frequently presents late with extensive florid callus, clinically and radiographically simulating osteogenic sarcoma

Ancillary aids

These patients need considerable encouragement to attain mobility. Essential in this is the provision of suitable walking aids, calipers and braces meticulously made and fitted. Children under five years are helped if knee hinges are omitted

FURTHER READING

Bannister, C.M. (1972) A method of repair of myelomeningoceles. *British Journal of Surgery,* **59**, 445-448.

Lorber, J. (1972) Spina bifida cystica. Results of treatment of 270 consecutive cases with criteria for selection for the future. *Archives of Disease in Childhood,* **47**, 854-873.

Sharrard, W.J.W. (1969) The orthopaedic surgery of cerebral palsy and spina bifida. In *Recent Advances in Orthopaedics.* First edn. ed. Apley A.G. London: Churchill.

Sharrard, W.J.W. & Drennan, J.C. (1972) Osteotomy-excision of the spine for lumbar kyphosis in older children with myelomeningocele. *Journal of Bone and Joint Surgery,* **54B**, 50-60.

Sharrard, W.J.W. & Grosfield, I. (1968) The management of deformity and paralysis of the foot in myelomeningocele. *Journal of Bone and Joint Surgery,* **50B**, 456-465.

Non-accidental injury in children

EXTENT OF PROBLEM

4,500 children in the United Kingdom per year are affected
Some estimate 10 to 17% die and 30% are permanently
handicapped

DIAGNOSTIC SUSPICION

1. Discrepancy between story and injuries
2. Delay in attendance
3. Abnormal parent attitudes
4. Social and marital problems
5. Recurrent attender
6. Patterns of injury
   Injuries of different ages in one patient
   Multiple bruises, especially if different ages
   Torn upper lip fraenum
   Fractures of ribs and clavicle in very young
   Sub-dural haematoma with retinal haemorrhage
   Burns distributed around body especially if very localised

DIAGNOSIS

Admit on suspicion
Obtain names and previous addresses of family, doctors
Social report
History of injury to siblings
Examine thoroughly, including photographs
X-ray at least all long bones and chest for variable age
fractures and periosteal reactions
Spiral fractures in the very young are especially suspicious
Exclude other pathology—blood picture, etc.

MANAGEMENT

Under directorship of paediatricians
Consult with other organisations and individuals—GP,
   social workers, health visitor, community physician,
   welfare organisations, especially NSPCC
Assess the home
Provide psychiatric aid to the parents
(Place of Safety Order) Children and Young Persons Act 1963
Criminal prosecution has no place in clinical management

FOLLOW-UP

Very close supervision by medical social workers and other agencies available

FURTHER READING
Cameron, J.M. (1970) The battered baby. *British Journal of Hospital Medicine,* **4,** 769-777.
Medical Practice, Contemporary themes (1973) Non-accidental injury in children. *British Medical Journal,* iv, 656-658.

Fat embolism

INCIDENCE

Clinical incidence is 1 to 2% in all bone trauma including bone surgery and perosseous venography. Necropsy incidence is almost 100%

Less commonly occurs in pancreatitis, osteomyelitis, diabetes, steroid therapy and burns

PATHOLOGY

Confusion is partly due to embolic effects in the brain and partly to hypoxaemia

Rash is due to embolism

Hypoxaemia is due to embolism in the lungs causing a ventilation/perfusion defect and to a local effect in the alveoli producing a diffusion defect

DIAGNOSIS

Earliest sign is a measured hypoxaemia
1. Clinical signs consist of:
   i. Confusion or alteration in conscious level
   ii. Pyrexia, tachypnoea, tachycardia
   iii. Petechial rash of skin, mucosae, fundi
   iv. Less commonly frank cyanosis and haemoptysis
2. Investigations:
   i. Chest radiograph in the severe case shows a 'snow storm' appearance
   ii. Blood gas measurement shows hypoxaemia
   iii. Radioactive lung scan shows multiple areas of loss of perfusion
   iv. Examination of sputum for fat—unreliable
   v. Examination of urine for fat—unreliable
   vi. Nephelometry gives a quantitative estimate of fat globules in plasma but is affected by other factors
   vii. Serum calcium is lowered in cases with poor prognosis

MANAGEMENT

1. Supportive:
    i.   Oxygen by mask or by tube depending on response assessed by blood gas measurement. May need ventilation with intermittent positive pressure and positive end expiratory pressure
    ii. Steroids
    iii. Antibiotics
2. Attempted specific therapies, not of proven value
    i.   Low molecular dextrans and alpha blockers
    ii. Clofibrate

O'Driscoll, M. & Powell, F.J. (1967) Injury, serum lipids, fat embolism and clofibrate. *British Medical Journal,* iv, 149-151.

    iii. Heparin
    iv. Pulmonary embolectomy—reported once in a severe case

Nelson, C.S. (1974) Cardiac and pulmonary fat embolectomy for suspected fat embolism. *Thorax,* **29,** 134-137.

FURTHER READING
Ross, A.P.J. (1970) The fat embolism syndrome. *Annals of the Royal College of Surgeons of England,* **46,** 159-171.

Low back syndromes

PRESENTATION

Symptoms may be due to:
  i. Compression or tethering of dura or neural tissue in the canal or foraminae
  ii. Degenerative disease of the facet joints
  iii. Inflammatory disease of the facet joints
  iv. Inflammatory disease of the disc or vertebral body
  v. Instability from any cause

Site of symptoms may be:
  i. Local
  ii. Referred due to nerve root compression—follows dermatome and somatotome pattern
  iii. Referred due to common innervation of structures—does not follow an obvious anatomical pattern

PATHOLOGY

Compression commonly due to:
  i. Disc degeneration
  ii. Facet osteophytes
  iii. Spondylolisthesis
  iv. The possibility of tumour must always be remembered

All causes of compression are more significant in the presence of spinal stenosis, either congenital or acquired due to degenerative disease

Instability commonly due to:
  i. Congenital anomaly
  ii. Degenerative disease
  iii. Fracture of the pars interarticularis
  iv. Ligamentous disruption from trauma

DIAGNOSIS
Based on:
   i.   History
   ii. Clinical examination
   iii. Plain radiographs

Further investigations include:
   i.   Tomography—linear and axial
   ii. Contrast radiography:
        a. Oil based myelography
        b. Air myelography
        c. Water-soluble medium radiculography
        d. Discography
   iii. Electrical conduction studies
   iv. Electromyography
   v.   'Pentothal studies'—study especially of straight leg
        raising response when recovering from general anaes-
        thetic

CONSERVATIVE MANAGEMENT
   i.   Rest
   ii. Rest plus traction
   iii. Local rest:
        a. Corsets and supports
        b. Plaster of Paris jackets
   iv. Analgesic and anti-inflammatory drugs
   v.   Physiotherapy:
        a. Traction—continuous
                    intermittent
        b. Exercises to strengthen back flexors, extensors and
           abdominals
        c. Manipulation
        d. Mobilisation of individual joints
        e. Heat in various forms—tends only to be temporary
           local palliative
   vi. Injections of local anaesthetic and hydrocortisone:
        a. To local tender spots
        b. To posterior primary ramus of nerve roots especially in
           facet arthropathy
        c. Epidural or caudal
   vii. Manipulation under anaesthetic

AIMS OF SURGERY
   i.   Decompression of spinal cord and/or nerve roots
   ii. Stabilisation of unstable segments and prevention of
        progression
   iii. Immobilisation of degenerate joints and discs

INDICATIONS FOR SURGERY
Compression syndromes
i.   Immediate:
     Disturbance of bladder function or rapidly progressive
     neurological loss
ii. Soon:
     Progressive motor loss in the lower limbs.
     Decompression is not often helpful in the presence of
     established motor loss
iii. Elective:
     Progression of the syndrome
     Failure to respond to conservative measures in the
     presence of neurological signs or severe symptoms.
     Recurrent incapacitating symptoms

Instability syndromes
i.   Symptomatic instability known to progress—due to
     congenital defects in the facet joints or due to defects in
     the pars interarticularis
ii. Symptomatic instability demonstrable radiographically
iii. Symptomatic instability due to degenerative disease in
     the facet joints. Fusion in such cases tends to be
     successful and give reliable long term results if the lesion
     is confined to one or two vertebral levels
Note that symptoms may be due to degenerative disease at a
level other than that which is unstable

SURGICAL MANAGEMENT
1. *Chemonucleolysis*
    Enzymatic destruction of a disc by an extract of papain,
    'Chymopapain'. Suitable particularly for a relatively recent
    disc prolapse. Complicated by a significant incidence of
    anaphylaxis
2. *Fenestration or hemilaminectomy with discectomy*
3. *Decompression procedures*
    i.   Total laminectomy
    ii. Decompression of the lateral recess by excision of facets
    iii. Deroofing of the root canal
         Such a procedure may need to be combined with fusion
         to avoid subsequent instability

4. Fusion

i.   Posterior—not often used since it makes later access to the canal very difficult and decorticating the laminae may induce hypertrophy and iatrogenic stenosis

ii.   Anterior—especially used for spondylolisthesis

iii.   Postero-lateral and intertransverse.
Very useful and may be performed without clearing the laminae at all

Wiltse, L.L., Bateman, J.G., Hutchinson, R.H. & Nelson, W.E. (1968) The paraspinal sacro-spinalis splitting approach to the lumbar spine. *Journal of Bone and Joint Surgery*, **50A**, 919-926.

iv.   Screw fusion across the facets

Boucher, H.H. (1959) A method of spinal fusion. *Journal of Bone and Joint Surgery*, **41B**, 248-259.

v.   Screw fusion across a defect in the pars interarticularis

Buck, J.E. (1970) Direct repair of the defect in spondylolisthesis. *Journal of Bone and Joint Surgery*, **52B**, 432-437.

Specifically used for spondylolisthesis due to that cause

FURTHER READING

Newman, P.H. (1973) Surgical treatment for derangement of the lumbar spine. *Journal of Bone and Joint Surgery*, **55B**, 7-19.

Sullivan, M.F. (1976) Low back pain. *British Journal of Hospital Medicine*, **15**, 25-36.

Symposium (1968) Low back pain and sciatic pain. *Journal of Bone and Joint Surgery*, **50A**, 166-210.

Causes of spinal cord compression

1. **Tumour, primary and secondary**
Intradural
   Extramedullary
      Neurofibroma
      Meningioma
      Dermoid
      Implantation dermoid from lumbar puncture
   Intramedullary
      Ependymoma
      Astrocytoma
Extradural
   Secondary carcinoma
   Primary bone tumour, especially myeloma
   Reticulosis
   Chordoma
   Neurofibroma
   Meningioma

2. **Infection**
Intradural
   Infected dermoid
   Tuberculoma
Extradural
   Pyogenic osteomyelitis or discitis
   Tuberculosis

3. **Arachnoid cysts—intermittent compression**

4. **Prolapsed intervertebral disc**

5. **Spinal injury**
   Compression by bone
   Compression by haematoma
   Haematomyelia

6. **Syringomyelia**

7. **Spondylolisthesis**

8.   Skeletal deformity
Kyphoscoliosis
Achondroplasia
Diastematomyelia
Spina bifida with lipoma

9.   Paget's disease

10. Hyperparathyroidism

Hall, A.J. & Mackay, N.N.S. (1973) The results of laminectomy for compression of the cord or cauda equina by extradural malignant tumour. *Journal of Bone and Joint Surgery,* **55B**, 497-505.

Harries, B. (1970) Spinal cord compression. *British Medical Journal,* i, 611-614, 673-676.

Osteomyelitis

BACTERIOLOGY

1. Neonates:
Staphylococcus predominates, about 95%
Streptococcus and gram-negative organisms are much less common

2. Children:
Staphylococcus is again the commonest
Tuberculous infection is usually secondary to tuberculous arthritis

3. Adults:
Commonest osteomyelitis arises as a direct result of open injury to the bone and many different organisms may be found
Infections with rarer organisms may present with infections of the vertebral column, e.g. brucella, pseudomonas, however the staphylococcus is the commonest organism.

NEONATAL OSTEOMYELITIS

1. Patients may present with septicaemia in which case a primary bone focus should be looked for
2. Treatment:
    i.   Should be early with massive doses of antibiotics once blood cultures have been taken
    ii. If not markedly improved at 12 to 24 hours from commencement of treatment the bone should be surgically drained since the whole diaphysis may become ischaemic from periosteal stripping by pus.
3. These children frequently form massive sequestra but with suitable protection from trauma they have extensive abilities to remodel and absorb the sequestum

ACUTE OSTEOMYELITIS IN THE OLDER AGE GROUP

There are two schools of thought for and against early surgery in acute osteomyelitis in limb bones

Advantages of early surgery
i.   Diagnosis is confirmed
ii. Pus is obtained for culture
iii. Early decompression is achieved and hence less risk of ischaemia

Disadvantages
  i.   Surgery is performed upon a very ill patient
  ii. Frequently operation is unnecessary for simple
       subperiosteal infection
  iii. Surgery, especially if combined with exploration of the
       medullary cavity, may spread a localised infection
Both regimes involve early treatment on suspicion of the
diagnosis with massive dosage of antibiotics. These are selected
on the basis of the known sensitivities of the staphylococcus in
the area until results from culture are obtained.
The conservative regime involves close supervision with
intervention if the patient fails to improve or shows a spread of
the disease process, e.g. a palpably increasing subperiosteal
abscess

CHRONIC OSTEOMYELITIS

Primary chronic osteomyelitis
  Presents with deep bone pain and a sclerotic cavity evident on
  radiographs
  Treated by surgical excision of the cavity leaving sloping
  margins to prevent further collections of pus.
  Traditionally this cavity is left to granulate and then lined with
  skin graft. With antibiotic cover the skin can usually be
  sutured primarily

Secondary chronic osteomyelitus
  Secondary either to trauma or to acute osteomyelitis
  If a sequestrum is present this may be removed but the main
  treatment is conservative with antibiotics for acute flare-ups.
  In some localised chronic osteomyelitis the area can be
  excised and saucerised

INFECTIONS OF THE VERTEBRAL COLUMN

Acute discitis and osteomyelitis rarely need surgery in the early stages unless the diagnosis is seriously in doubt or there is evidence of neurological involvement.

Surgery in the presence of established paraplegia is rarely helpful.

In the early stages tuberculosis may be managed with chemotherapy alone. An MRC trial is showing some good results even in established tuberculous osteomyelitis

Medical Research Council Working Party on tuberculosis of the spine (1973) A controlled trial of ambulant out-patient treatment and in-patient rest in the management of tuberculosis of the spine in young Korean patients on standard chemotherapy. *Journal of Bone and Joint Surgery,* **55B,** 678-697.

Medical Research Council Working Party on tuberculosis of the spine (1973) A controlled trial of plaster-of-Paris jackets in the management of ambulant out-patient treatment of tuberculosis of the spine in children on standard chemotherapy. A study in Pusan, Korea. *Tubercle,* **54,** 261-282.

If there is a large area of involvement, with bone destruction, then decompression and bone grafting is required.

FURTHER READING

British Medical Journal (1972) Some problems of acute osteomyelitis. *British Medical Journal,* iv, 317.

Blockey, N.J. & McAllister, T.A. (1972) Antibiotics in acute osteomyelitis in children. *Journal of Bone and Joint Surgery,* **54B,** 299-309.

Trueta, J. (1959) The three types of acute haematogenous osteomyelitis. *Journal of Bone and Joint Surgery,* **41B,** 671-680.

Internal fixation in fracture surgery

PRINCIPLES OF INTERNAL FIXATION
1. Knowledge of the anatomy and physiology of the parts
2. Surgical technique with minimum of soft tissue disturbance
3. Primary object is bony union and restoration of function
4. Early mobilisation of the part

INDICATIONS
1. Failure to maintain or achieve adequate reduction of fracture
2. Need for early mobilisation of the part or patient
3. Soft tissue complications—vascular, neurological
4. Other need for open operation—bone grafting, osteotomy, arthrodesis
5. Need for very accurate anatomical reduction, e.g. Bennett's, some Pott's, fractures
6. Multiple fractures in one bone or leg
7. Pathological fracture

Fidler, M. (1973) Prophylactic internal fixation of secondary neoplastic deposits in long bones. *British Medical Journal,* i, 341-343.

CONTRAINDICATIONS
1. Compound fracture—relative contraindication since soft tissues may heal better over rigidly fixed bone
2. Previous infection—again relative

MEANS USED
1. Wires—Kirschner, cerclage, figure of eight
2. Applied—screws, plates, staples
3. Intramedullary—Kuntscher, Rush nails
4. Combinations—nail plates, Y-nail

PRINCIPLES OF COMPRESSION TECHNIQUES
Rigid fixation leads to bone repair at right angles to shaft
Rigid fixation plus compression leads to primary endosteal union with minimal callus—'primary bone union'.

Compression techniques
1. Interfragmental:
    a. Lag screws with length of plain shank
    b. Lag effect with fully threaded screws by over-drilling the proximal bone
2. Axial:
    Achieved by compression on the side under distraction force—tension band principle
3. Combination of interfragmental compression with plate neutralisation of rotational forces
4. Intramedullary fixation plus weight-bearing

Müller, M.E., Allgower, M. & Willenegger, H. (1970) *Manual of Internal Fixation.* Berlin: Springer-Verlag.

Complications
1. Infection
2. Metal fatigue—mechanical failure
3. Loss of bone resilience
4. Change in bone architecture leading to weakness
5. Additional muscle adhesions from surgery

FURTHER READING
Cockin, J. (1973) Advances in the operative treatment of fractures. *British Journal of Hospital Medicine,* **10**, 744-750.
McNeur, J.C. (1970) The management of open skeletal trauma with particular reference to internal fixation. *Journal of Bone and Joint Surgery,* **52B**, 54-60.
Sevitt, S. (1970) Bone repair and fracture healing. *British Journal of Hospital Medicine,* **3**, 693-710.

Osteotomy

AIMS OF PROCEDURE

1. To correct deformities—congenital or acquired
2. To realign joints:
   To prevent degeneration
   To slow degeneration
   To aid remodelling of bones
   To give greater stability
3. To relieve pain
4. To aid repair of fractures

First metatarsal

1. Indications

Hallux valgus due to metatarsus primus varus

2. Techniques

i. Distal transverse osteotomies of various kinds leaving small pegs for fixation into the medulla of the displaced portion. Technically can be difficult
ii. Proximal wedge osteotomies, there is little cancellous bone here and therefore is prone to non-union
iii. Distal oblique osteotomy sliding the distal portion proximally and medially. May be simply held with plaster

3. Mechanism

i. Realignment of the metatarsal
ii. Realignment of tendons

Knee

1. Indications

i. Osteo-arthrosis of mild to moderate degree especially if affecting one compartment more than the other
ii. Rheumatoid arthritis in fairly early stage

2. Techniques

i. Wedge osteotomies. Usually performed in upper tibia above the tibial tuberosity in an area of good cancellous bone. Particularly useful if there is varus or valgus deformity but requires accurate preoperative measurement of the angle required and accurate cutting at operation.
ii. Bracket osteotomy. An inverted-U shaped osteotomy performed above the tibial tuberosity and varus or valgus corrected by eye on the table, the corrected position being maintained by stepped staples or compression pins

iii.   Double osteotomy. Subarticular osteotomy of tibia with osteotomy of the femoral condyles at the level of the top of the articular surface parallel to the floor (on standing) Postoperatively walking in a plaster of Paris cylinder until six weeks when a manipulation under anaesthetic may be required

Benjamin, A.J. (1969) Double osteotomy for the painful knee in rheumatoid and osteoarthritis. *Journal of Bone and Joint Surgery,* **51B**, 694-699.

3. Mechanism
i.   Realignment of line of weight bearing
ii.   Non-specific 'osteotomy effect' attributed to:
    a.   Relief of pressure in medullary cavity
    b.   Change in vascularity due to bone repair
    c.   Change in neural innervation of the joint
    d.   Non-specific changes in bony architecture due to fracture and repair

Neck of femur
1. Indications
i.   Early osteo-arthrosis with severe symptoms but a good range of movement
ii.   To correct deformity—varus, valgus or rotation
iii. To correct lack of cover of the femoral head in the presence of early degeneration
iv.   To correct the deformity of slipped upper femoral epiphysis and encourage union
v.   To control remodelling in Perthes' disease
vi.   To ensure congruent reduction of the hip in congenital dislocation or acetabular dysplasia
vii. To encourage union of an ununited fracture neck of femur, especially the subcapital type
2. Techniques
i.   With very few exceptions the osteotomy is usually performed at the level of, or just below, the lesser trochanter
ii.   With a laterally based or medially based wedge to correct varus or valgus respectively
iii. With or without rotation
iv.   With or without medial displacement of the distal portion. This realigns weightbearing and also ensures a richer blood supply around the neck of the femur
v.   With or without internal fixation. Nail plate or one piece spline with or without compression

3. *Mechanism*
    i.   In osteoarthrosis:
         a.   Change of line of loadbearing
         b.   'Osteotomy effect'
         c.   Stimulates soft tissue cover of the femoral head
    ii. In Perthes' disease:
         In congenital dislocation of the hip and acetabular dysplasia it has been shown that the modelling of the femoral head and acetabulum is due to the mutual counter-pressure between the surfaces.
         The accuracy of the final anatomical modelling is due to the congruency of these surfaces; this congruency may be achieved by osteotomy
    iii. In ununited fractures of neck of femur osteotomy stimulates the development of hyperaemia around the fracture site

Pelvis
1. *Indications*
    i.   Maintain reduction of congenitally dislocated hip
    ii. Aid remodelling in acetabular dysplasia and Perthes' disease
    iii. Improve the cover or congruency of the femoral head in established degrees of acetabular dysplasia with early symptomatic degenerative disease
2. *Techniques*
    i.   Salter—innominate osteotomy performed from the greater sciatic notch to above the acetabulum then tilting the acetabular portion downwards and outwards securing the final position with a wedge shaped bone graft from the iliac crest.

Salter, R.B. (1966) Role of innominate osteotomy in the treatment of congenital dislocation and subluxation of the hip in the older child. *Journal of Bone and Joint Surgery,* **48A**, 1413-1439.

    ii. Chiari—osteotomy immediately above the superior lip of the acetabulum displacing the acetabulum medially, thereby producing a prolongation of the acetabulum laterally

Arthroplasty

TYPES OF ARTHROPLASTY
   i.   Excision
   ii. Insertion of a liner or spacer into the joint
   iii. Replacement of one surface of the joint
   iv. Total replacement

IDEAL REPLACEMENT ARTHROPLASTY
   i.   Gives pain relief
   ii. Is capable of bearing the load required
   iii. Gives an adequate range of movement
   iv. Materials are compatible with the tissues in both the formed and wear product state
   v. Low wear rate leading to a long duration of life
   vi. Low coefficient of friction

In practice there are very many different designs each with different claimed advantages

INDICATIONS FOR ARTHROPLASTY
   i.   Primarily pain
   ii. Occasionally stiffness
   iii. As an adjunct to correction of deformity in association with joint pathology
   iv. Following trauma particularly to neck of femur

COMPLICATIONS OF REPLACEMENT ARTHROPLASTIES
   i.   Infection
   ii. Loosening of components
   iii. Breaking of components
   iv. Metal sensitivity
   v. Oncogenesis demonstrated in animals

Swanson, S.A.V., Freeman, M.A.R. & Heath, J.C. (1973) Laboratory tests on total joint replacement prostheses. *Journal of Bone and Joint Surgery*, **55B**, 759-773.

INDIVIDUAL JOINTS

1. Fingers

i.   Proximal interphalangeal joint, rarely indicated, either metal hinge or elastomer

ii. Metacarpophalangeal joint, hinge or elastomer flexible spacer. When used for rheumatoid arthritis usually needs to be associated with careful tendon balancing and soft tissue correction.
Problems—some spacers have snapped but in the presence of good balancing they may not need to be replaced

2. Carpus

i.   Excision of individual bones especially trapezium for osteo-arthrosis and lunate or scaphoid for symptomatic non-union or necrosis

ii. Excision of entire proximal row for grossly degenerate and subluxed wrist where arthrodesis is not indicated

iii. Insertion of plastic and elastomer sheeting in the joint space has been tried with mixed results

iv. Replacement of individual bones with a spacer
Problem with spacers has been in fixation in the carpus. The trapezium is fixed to the base of the first metacarpal

3. Distal radio-ulnar joint

i.   Excision of distal end of ulna

ii. Replacement of distal end of ulna with a spacer

4. Proximal radio-ulnar joint

i.   Excision of head of radius

ii. Replacement of head of radius with a spacer

5. Elbow

Excision arthroplasty of the elbow can restore some useful function particularly in the presence of extensive scarring after trauma or infection
Replacement by hinge prostheses is performed
Problems: designing an adequate form of fixation is difficult and many prostheses have become loose with time

6. Shoulder

i.   Excision unless associated with very extensive fibrosis tends to lead to a useless flail arm

ii. Hemireplacement—replacement of the head of the humerus is occasionally necessary for fractures of the head and neck where the articular surface is avascular or the fracture is very comminuted

iii. Total replacement—a number of designs are still in the
    trial stages
    Problems:
  a. It is difficult to obtain secure fixation to the glenoid
  b. The prosthesis is subject to distraction stresses when
     carrying loads and subject to load bearing stresses
     when using a stick or crutches
  c. There tends to be a poor range of movement after
     replacement due to the fixed axis of rotation of the
     prosthesis compared to the sliding axis in the normal
     shoulder
  d. Patients with shoulders needing replacement tend to
     have poor muscular control of the shoulder

7. Foot
  i. Excision:
    a. First proximal phalanx base for hallux valgus
    b. Other proximal phalanges for subluxed claw toes
    c. Heads of metatarsals for disorganised
      metatarsophalangeal joints
  ii. Replacement—occasionally a spacer is inserted to
    replace the base of the first proximal phalanx

8. Ankle
Replacement is rarely indicated since arthrodesis is so
effective. Total replacement has been devised for the talo-
tibial joint

9. Knee
  i. Hemireplacement: replacement of one or both tibial
    articular surfaces with metal
    Indications:
    a. Monocompartmental osteo-arthrosis
    b. Mild to moderate osteo-arthrosis with marked
      symptoms
    Problems:
Fixation can be difficult and if inadequate the plates can
sublux.

ii.   Hinge replacement: may be metal to metal joint or may include high density polyethylene bushes to reduce friction
Problems:
a.   Some designs need large bone resection making subsequent arthrodesis if required difficult
b.   Fixed axis of rotation prevents rotation and loosening of the stems may occur from high torque strains
Advantages:
a.   Good early postoperative movement
b.   Stable knee

iii. Two-part replacement: one piece of metal replacing the femoral condyles which may or may not include a slot to permit retention of the cruciate ligaments; one (or two) pieces of polyethylene replacing the tibial surface.
Problems:
May have poor stability if there is ligamentous damage.
Advantages:
a.   Sliding axis of rotation in flexion
b.   Permits rotation at the knee
c.   Fairly small bone resection rendering subsequent arthrodesis if required easier
To give greater stability some of these prostheses are now partially constrained either by the geometry of their design or by a loose link between the components.

Attenborough, C.G. (1976) Total knee replacement using the stabilised gliding prosthesis. *Annals of the Royal College of Surgeons of England.* **58**, 1, 4-14

iv.   Four-part replacement: two metal femoral 'wheels' articulating with two polyethylene tibial 'tracks'. The wheels are constructed with differing geometry in different designs
Problems:
a.   Require very accurate surgical technique
b.   Very small surface area of load bearing and of fixation to bone
Advantages:
a.   Preserves all ligaments giving greater stability
b.   Minimal bone resection permitting simple arthrodesis if required

10. Hip
Most frequently performed arthroplasty
i.   Excision: occasionally performed in presence of severe deformity, e.g. long standing congenital dislocation of the hip with degeneration. Most frequently seen now as the end result of a 'failed' total replacement arthroplasty
ii.   Insertion of a liner: cup arthroplasty, occasionally performed in young patients with hip degeneration

iii. Hemireplacement: replacement of the femoral head, occasionally performed for degenerative disease but most frequently for subcapital fracture of the neck of the femur in the elderly

iv. Total replacement: most designs are two part with a metal or polyethylene acetabular component and a metal femoral component. A few designs are for use without cement, most are designed to be inserted with bone cement (polymethyl methacrylate)

    a. Very many designs, about 400

    b. Main problem is infection since this almost entirely precludes further replacement

       Ultra-clean theatre techniques may reduce this problem

    c. Metal allergy, especially to nickel and cobalt, has been implicated as a cause of loosening

Evans, E.M., Miller, A.J. & Vernon-Roberts, B. (1974) Metal sensitivity as a cause of bone necrosis and loosening of the prosthesis in total joint replacement. *Journal of Bone and Joint Surgery*, **56B**, 626-642.

    d. Technique of insertion is important since small errors of position lead to dislocation

CONSIDERATIONS IN THE SELECTION OF HIP PROSTHESES

1. Materials

i. Metal on plastic results in:

    a. Decreased friction

    b. Decreased metal wear products

    c. Decreased wear resistance compared to metal on metal

ii. Stainless steel in the fully softened state is:

    a. Very corrosion resistant

    b. Readily forged in manufacture

    c. Relatively cheap

    d. Relatively low in tensile strength

       Non-softened stainless steel is slightly less corrosion resistant but has a much greater tensile strength

iii. Cobalt/chrome alloy is:

    a. Very corrosion resistant

    b. Manufactured by casting

    c. Expensive

    d. Relatively high in tensile strength

       The castings are more uniform in quality if vacuum melt/vacuum cast techniques are used but this is expensive

iv. Titanium [318] (alloy with vanadium and aluminium) is:

    a. Expensive

    b. Poor in wear resistance unless anodised

    c. Used in presence of known metal allergy

2. Design

i. A small head results in:
   a. Less friction
   b. Probably less wear products
   c. Increased load/surface area
   d. Increased rate of depth of wear

ii. Shape of shaft affects:
   a. Ease of insertion
   b. Resistance to fatigue failure
   c. Line of load bearing

iii. Length of shaft affects:
   a. Load/area ratio
   b. Area of contact with cement
   c. Extent to which the bow of the femur affects rotation of the prosthesis

iv. Length of neck determines:
   a. Line of load bearing
   b. Clearance of bony surfaces for movement

FURTHER READING

British Medical Journal (1975) Rises and uses of total hip replacement. *British Medical Journal,* ii, 296.

Dee, R. (1972) Total replacement arthroplasty of the elbow for rheumatoid arthritis. *Journal of Bone and Joint Surgery,* **54B**, 88-95.

Potter, T.A., Wainfield, M.S. & Thomas, W.H. (1972) Arthroplasty of the knee. *Journal of Bone and Joint Surgery,* **54A**, 1-24.

Swanson, A.B. (1972) Flexible implant arthroplasty for arthritic finger joints. *Journal of Bone and Joint Surgery,* **54A**, 435-455.

These are illustrative articles only, there are many more on differing prostheses.